Common Immunity

Common Immunity

Biopolitics in the Age of the Pandemic

Roberto Esposito

Translated by Zakiya Hanafi

polity

First published in Italian as *Immunità comune. Biopolitica all'epoca della pandemia* © 2022 Giulio Einaudi editore s.p.a., Torino

This English edition © Polity Press, 2023

This book has been translated thanks to a translation grant awarded by the Italian Ministry of Foreign Affairs and International Cooperation / Questo libro è stato tradotto grazie a un contributo alla traduzione assegnato dal Ministero degli Affari Esteri e della Cooperazione Internazionale italiano.

Polity Press
65 Bridge Street
Cambridge CB2 1UR, UK

Polity Press
111 River Street
Hoboken, NJ 07030, USA

ISBN-13: 978-1-5095-5564-2 – hardback
ISBN-13: 978-1-5095-5565-9 – paperback

A catalogue record for this book is available from the British Library.

Library of Congress Control Number: 2022948118

Typeset in 11 on 13pt Sabon by
Cheshire Typesetting Ltd, Cuddington, Cheshire

Printed and bound in Great Britain by CPI Group (UK) Ltd, Croydon

The publisher has used its best endeavours to ensure that the URLs for external websites referred to in this book are correct and active at the time of going to press. However, the publisher has no responsibility for the websites and can make no guarantee that a site will remain live or that the content is or will remain appropriate.

Every effort has been made to trace all copyright holders, but if any have been overlooked the publisher will be pleased to include any necessary credits in any subsequent reprint or edition.

For further information on Polity, visit our website:
politybooks.com

Contents

Acknowledgment

The English edition of this book was prepared with remarkable alacrity and accuracy thanks, in part, to the keen eye and dedication of researcher and copyeditor Manuela Tecusan.

Introduction

1

The Great Barrington Declaration, named after the town in Massachusetts where it was drafted, was published on October 5, 2020. Promoted by a think tank that defines itself as "libertarian," the Declaration is actually part of a right-wing American network that has gone so far as to deny the climate emergency, in line with the politics of the former president, Donald Trump (who lost no time in endorsing it). In the Declaration, several virologists take a stand in favor of "herd immunity," in opposition to the policies adopted by most European governments during the pandemic phase. Arguing that these policies produce devastating effects on public health – a decrease in childhood vaccinations and cancer screenings, an increase in cardiovascular diseases, and a deterioration of mental health – the Declaration intends "to minimize mortality and social harm until we reach herd immunity."[1] The supposed advantage of this approach would be that young people and adults in good health are allowed to live normally, while those who are most vulnerable by reason of age and state of health are isolated. The approach is premised on the belief that society as a whole will be protected because, as the rate of natural immunity from infection rises, the virus will eventually die out, having nowhere left to spread. This strategy of "focused protection" intends to keep schools, universities, businesses, and cultural centers open, relying on the rapid spread of infection to reach the kind of immunization that would protect even the frailest.

Defined as "ridiculous" by Anthony Fauci, the doyen of American epidemiologists, in a matter of days the Declaration was harshly criticized in the John Snow Memorandum – an open letter published in the *Lancet* by eighty specialists in infectious diseases and health systems. In their view, the Great Barrington Declaration is nothing but "a dangerous fallacy unsupported by scientific evidence," since "any pandemic management strategy relying upon immunity from natural infections for COVID-19 is flawed."[2] Not only would it have lethal effects on the entire population, it would also worsen the inequalities already laid bare by the pandemic – and with negative medical and social consequences. The John Snow Memorandum categorically denies the idea that an immunity produced through infection instead of vaccination can end the pandemic. Immunity from infection would not only fail to achieve this result, but it would also create a huge number of victims. Furthermore, compulsory confinement of the most vulnerable swathes of population "is practically impossible and highly unethical," because it would condemn one section of the population to forced isolation while exposing the other to unpredictable consequences for health. The only acceptable way forward is to extend protection to the whole society by interrupting the chain of infection through general measures of confinement and distancing. Restriction of movements, mass testing, and contact tracing are the only adequate strategy for stopping the progress of the virus, or at least slowing it down, while waiting for the vaccine to weaken it. These are the exact measures adopted, sometimes after rapid policy reversals, by almost all the countries touched by the pandemic.

As we know, this alternative was implemented in dramatic fashion during the first phase but was later superseded by the production and distribution of vaccines on a vast scale. The aim was to achieve a generalized immunity, which would be due this time to vaccine prevention rather than to infection. We know that this third response – the only one that is scientifically reliable and, until proven otherwise, effective – has also met with uneven success. Competition between vaccines, the shortage of available supplies in the face of demand, miscommunications regarding their different safety and efficacy – not to mention resistance from significant segments of the population that are hostile to vaccination – have complicated and delayed the immunization process. Without stopping it, though. Despite the explosion of successive variants with different degrees of vaccine resistance, no other avenue for fighting the disease has appeared, except to ramp up vaccine production as much as possible, through more and more advanced technologies. The number of doses that will be needed, who will be eligible for them, and at what price remains uncertain for the time being. Equally uncertain is how the battle will play out to waive patent protections and to liberalize vaccine licensure, actions to which big pharma is naturally opposed. The business these strategies seek to control is not related solely to healthcare: the industry also holds a strategic role in globally reshaping a new geopolitical balance of power.

We will discuss all this in the final pages of the book. But, before we get to that, let us pause over a more general consideration, which concerns its object and overall perspective. It can hardly escape notice that all three proposed solutions – natural herd immunity, social confinement, and generalized vaccination – are different modes of the immune paradigm, in which they all partake. The necessity for immunization, taken for granted by all parties in this dispute, is never in question; only its interpretation and implementation are. Should immunity be natural or induced, individual or collective, temporary or definitive? In a field that has become dominated entirely by the lexicon of immunization, these are the only open questions that remain. If the dynamics of immunization were already set into motion by the biopolitical regime under which we have lived for a long time, the arrival of the coronavirus simply picked up their pace to an extraordinary degree. All the proposals for combatting it that were made during the last year are simply different shades of the same immune syndrome, at once biological, legal, political, and technological. The measures taken by the various governments stand at the intersection of law and medicine, according to the bivalent meaning assumed by the concept of "security." During a pandemic, no security is more important than health security. But health security hinges on compliance with legally sanctioned norms. This is why biology and legal practice have become two sides of the same demand for security, which makes one the precondition of the other.

2

These ideas, which I presented in a book called *Immunitas: The Protection and Negation of Life*,[3] have been validated, down to their details, some twenty years later. This is hardly a source of personal satisfaction, given that the validation coincides with the most serious planetary crisis since the end of World War II. But contemporary society's propensity to immunize itself has certainly exceeded all imagination, becoming the most significant phenomenon of our time. For this very reason, then, it should not be examined *en bloc*, but rather broken down into types of different intensity and outcome. As regards, for example, the three alternatives mentioned earlier, their different statuses and effects must be acknowledged. Even though all three lie on the same immune horizon, they depart considerably from one another, both through their scientific premises and in their ethical protocols. The herd immunity advanced at the beginning of the pandemic in the United Kingdom, Sweden, the United States, and Brazil is based on thanatopolitical principles that foresee, if not the elimination, at least the marginalization of "less adapted" individuals, to the benefit of the more productive segments of the population. Conversely, protection through distancing, implemented by most governments before vaccination was available, is a negative biopolitical choice, because it ensures social protection through desocialization. Despite obvious difficulties in getting it off the ground and disseminating it, the third approach, if extended to the global community, is the only one that offers an affirmative biopolitics – one in which, for the first time in history, we can glimpse the unprecedented silhouette of a *common immunity*.

To arrive at it we must go through a few different but interrelated steps. The first concerns the paradigmatic relationship between the notions of community and immunity. They appear inseparable from the outset, both logically – since one is carved out of the other's negative space – and historically. There is no such thing as a community that lacks immune *dispositifs*. Without some sort of protective system to ensure permanence in time, no social body can withstand the conflicts that course through it over time, just as no human body can. Everything hinges on preserving an equilibrium that contains the social body within boundaries compatible with the society that the protective system seeks to preserve. Overstepping those boundaries, like a sort of autoimmune disease, risks provoking its collapse. In Covid-19, as we know, the immune system itself is responsible for the body's destructive inflammation, caused by an excessive response to the attack of the virus, a response destined to reproduce that attack in amplified form. But if this case is, like others, one of limiting an otherwise necessary device, how does one go about identifying it? On what does its preservation depend? And why is it so difficult to keep it under control?

The answers that this book provides concern the problematic relationship between the two sides of immunity: the legal–political and the medical–biological. Today immunity belongs to both vocabularies, converging in an idea of security that is at once medical and social. However, the semantic plexus that appears to us now as a single thing is the effect of an articulation between two meanings that for a long time remained distinct. Only in the last two centuries – since the discovery of such a thing as biological immunity – have they overlapped. Before then, for at least two thousand years, the largely prevalent side of immunity was the legal–political, in a sense not all that different from the meaning it holds today for diplomats and people whose professional dealings are protected from the general law. Apart from a few early literary metaphors, the biological meaning of the immune system, at least in a scientific understanding, remained muted for a long time. Such a delay explains why, when it appeared, it was immediately influenced by the legal–political interpretation of the term. This conditioned its definition, orienting it toward a meaning related to defense of the body – political, and even military – against external invaders. This conceptual shift from politics to medicine had two significant effects on how the immune system was understood, overshadowing its complex structure in favor of a more schematic picture that, in some ways, still holds the field, having been called into question only in the past fifty years.

The prevalence of the legal–political over the biomedical side applies to the theoretical level of the concepts but not to the historical reality, of course: the functioning of biological immunity is as old as humans, and in some way even predates them. From this point of view, the relations between the two sides are inverted. It was biological immunity, stronger or weaker depending on physiological and environmental circumstances, that conditioned political and military history. Right from the first wars of humankind and up to World War I, immune resistance, the ability, that is, to withstand destructive epidemics, played a decisive role in power relations between civilizations when they came into contact at certain points. The history of the conquest of America, which I examine in the first chapter, is a striking example of the importance that immunity – or lack of it – has played in the political and military balances of human history. Immunity has made it possible for a handful of determined men to take possession of vast empires. But there is something else this book sheds light on in the relationship between immunity and war: the fact that the discovery of vaccines, from Jenner's primitive variety to Pasteur's specific one, was itself a battle between national interests – a way of doing politics by means of medicine. "Pasteurism," the formidable healthcare machine that spread from the Pasteur Institute throughout France and then to the colonies – played a major role in this dialectic. The movement unfolded as a zero-sum clash between humans and bacteria, fought at the crossroads between healthcare practice and colonial expansion. The culmination of this twofold process of politicizing medicine and medicalizing politics took place in the no-holds-barred conflict that made adversaries of the two great "microbe hunters": Pasteur and Koch. Their confrontation in the scientific domain mirrored the hegemonic clash between France and Germany, along a thread that connects the Franco-Prussian War of 1870 to World War I.

3

The current biopolitical – or, more accurately perhaps, immuno-political – turn is examined in this book from two different but ultimately converging angles. The first concerns democracy, rightly defined as "immunitarian" by reason of the self-protective and at times exclusionary form it takes in relation to those whose equality it presupposes and yet does not recognize. The growing gap between segments unequal in terms of social and civil rights gives shape to a post-democratic regime that bears little more than the name of democracy. Such a discrepancy, now visible to the naked eye, is actually the result of a contradiction in the concept that has permeated democracy from the beginning, putting it at odds with itself. In democracy it would seem that freedom and equality, representation and identity, power and participation never come into balance, moving further and further apart. This is the source of the disbandment – highlighted by classical and contemporary interpreters – between the internally contradictory poles of an aristocratic democracy and a democratic despotism. By now it is clear that this contention cannot be resolved through mere formal adjustments: it calls for an institutional change that goes beyond the sphere of the sovereign state and engages more deeply with the social dynamic and its conflicts. From this point of view, contemporary democracy appears to be at a fork in the road that it can no longer avoid. Either it resigns itself to the autoimmune syndrome that some have predicted as a sort of destiny, or it must rethink all its institutions – and itself as an institution – in a form that puts the political battle, currently suffocated by the double incumbrance of the economy and technology, back into play.

The other issue this book explores is the interpretation of biopolitics itself. The jumble of criticisms devoid of argumentative substance that target this concept may come as a surprise – although not a big one to those who are familiar with these reactive dynamics – especially at a time when biopolitics has been irrefutably validated by the pandemic and the response to it in healthcare and other sectors. Events have substantiated and even surpassed Foucault's insights with disconcerting punctuality: medicalization of society, control over individuals and populations, deployment of governments' pastoral power – not to mention the generalization of the immune *dispositifs* mentioned earlier. Of course, we cannot embrace Foucault's biopolitics in totality: it was developed in a period different from our own, and it is not without its uncertainties and contradictions. Our task – to which these pages seek to contribute

– is to integrate his biopolitics and adapt it to a contemporary condition that he could not foresee, but to do it from an adequate understanding of his work. Perhaps the biggest misunderstanding that Foucault's critics fall into is that of accusing him of a naturalist or biologist reading, that is, of an ahistorical interpretation of "life" – which, on the contrary, he always intended in a deeply historical way. His 1976 course at the Collège de France, "Society Must Be Defended," is absolutely explicit on this point. True, the two later courses, "Security, Territory, Population" and "The Birth of Biopolitics," are oriented in a slightly different direction, focused as they are on the notion of economic government, which does not lend an affirmative character to the paradigm of biopolitics. One almost gets the impression that Foucault's discourse, in default of answers to its own questions, at a certain point folds in on itself. Here again, one of the reasons for this hermeneutic block could be that the concept of institution was not adequately developed. Although Foucault paid constant attention to it, his efforts were directed to bringing out its repressive side more than its potentially innovative aspects. From this perspective, too, the pandemic has given the theory a push forward, by shining a spotlight on the irreplaceable role of institutions and the need to transform them. What emerges from this is the necessity to rebuild a relationship between biopolitics and institutionalism that has thus far been impeded by an inadequate interpretation of both.

4

For now, let us turn our attention to the relationship between immunity and philosophy. The fact that it has only recently become an established scholarly focus should not cast its genealogy into oblivion. Even when twentieth-century thinkers do not address the immune paradigm directly – as in the case of Heidegger and Freud – the boldness with which its silhouette appears between the lines places it at the heart of modernization itself, and thus not as an alternative to the great interpretations of modernity (Max Weber's rationalization, Karl Löwith's secularization, Hans Blumenberg's self-legitimization), but in productive tension with them. My impression – to be verified, of course, by a longue durée study of the philosophical, literary, and anthropological sources – is that the founding texts of modernity, if read in a certain light, attest to the more or less recognizable presence of the immune *dispositif* as their general horizon of meaning. If this is true – if immunization turns out to be the secret name of civilization – it would mean that political ontology should not be understood as one particular rubric of knowledge or western power but as the deep web in which knowledge and power are embedded and that alone makes them recognizable.

Other authors, whom I also discuss in chapter 4, deal more openly with the issue of immunity, generally without referring to one another. My aim is to reconnect these threads by recovering their links in texts from varied lexical fields, which range from philosophy to psychoanalysis, sociology, and anthropology. From Nietzsche to Girard, from Luhmann to Sloterdijk, and up to Derrida, the immune paradigm is probed from different perspectives that appear to intersect at a point that gets concealed, and sometimes effaced, by the specialized languages these authors use. Without distorting their paths, I have sought to retrace the immune paradigm in a complex interplay with the concept of negativity. Already recognizable in Heidegger, especially in what he calls the reduction of the modern world to a picture and in the reassuring sense of "securedness" that the subject derives from it, the immune paradigm is presented by Freud in all the possible shades that, taken together, evoke the "discontents" of civilization. Civilization, required to dominate the hostile forces of nature, creates a malaise proportional to the inhibition of the erotic and aggressive drives of the subjects who experience it. But the negative, in the form of a lesser evil destined to protect us from a greater one, is the focal point of all the authors examined here. For Nietzsche, who interprets all modern institutions of knowledge and power as cogs in a single immune machine, life, which coincides with the will to power, requires a restraint capable of saving it from its own excess. From this point of view, immunization reveals itself as a negation of life that is necessary for life's facilitated survival. Like the Pauline figure of the *katechon*, it protects from evil by incorporating rather than excluding it.

According to René Girard and going along a path that follows and simultaneously criticizes the Freudian analytical framework, communities can protect themselves from the violence that courses through them only by directing it onto a sacrificial victim that draws all violence onto itself – until a messiah offers himself spontaneously to death, revealing, and thereby deactivating, the sacrificial mechanism. Central to this mechanism is the law, which secularizes the sacrificial paradigm but does not eliminate it, using violence to immunize society from violence, on which it claims a monopoly. It is striking that Niklas Luhmann, while adopting a less radical theoretical position, nevertheless identifies the law as the immune subsystem of social systems. Moreover, from the perspective of a communication identified with immunization, he acknowledges that the system functions only through the use of "noes" – contradictions, that is, that put society in a state of alert, thus saving it from unsustainable conflicts. But it is Jacques Derrida and Peter Sloterdijk who, from different directions, engage directly with the issue of immunity. Derrida does so through autoimmune words that express the suicidal process of the immune system against the body politic that this system nevertheless defends, contradictorily. Democracy can therefore safeguard itself only by negating itself, or at least by suspending itself in a form that goes against its own values. Sloterdijk creates a true social immunology, constructed along vertical lines that follow the passage of time and along horizontal lines in the globalized dimension of space. What is even more striking is that both philosophers, albeit starting from very distant premises, search in the autoimmunization of immunity for the future profile of an unprecedented "co-immunity."

5

The last chapter of the book connects these historical and conceptual investigations to the frightful yet illuminating years of our current period. When not intended to create panic, the terrifying predictions of novels, films, and pandemic scenarios, but also the catastrophic forecasts of some scientists, all of which seemed exaggerated, proved to be largely realistic and even understated by comparison with what took place between 2020 and 2021. Reductionist, if not conspiratorial interpretations of the ongoing pandemic quickly crumbled in the face of millions of deaths worldwide. Already in the spring of last year it became apparent to anyone with a grain of commonsense that these ideas were simply wrong – not because they highlighted potential deviations of the immune paradigm, which has since entered the distinctive lexicon of our time, but because they lost sight of its inner complexity, its simultaneously necessary and dangerous character. "Necessary" because, more than ever before, the only possible prospect of defense for a devastating viral disease such as this one is immunization, in its various forms. "Dangerous" because its escalation can give rise to the perverse effects that we have experienced on more than one occasion. What governments have often missed in their pandemic policies – putting aside assessment and implementation errors, delays, failures to act, and contradictions – is the ability to discern and distinguish between protective and constrictive modes of individual and collective life.

In this book, all the issues at stake – the relationship between the right to life and the right to freedom, between state of exception and state of emergency, between science, technology, and politics, between competition and disparity in vaccine acquisition – are grouped under the immune paradigm, which one way or another forms the horizon of their meaning. The pandemic accelerated the connection between technization and immunization that has been underway for some time, objectively weakening the political sphere. The figure of the expert – not always coincident with that of the scientist – has assumed a somewhat disturbing prominence in this context, often predetermining the space for political decision-making, which is inevitably depoliticized as a result. Despite a pervasive formulaic image, technocracy is not the opposite of populism but rather one of its equally insidious faces, to which the only non-regressive response is an affirmative biopolitics. This, of course, is a narrow passage to navigate, made even more difficult by the pandemic, although – and this thesis underlies the entire book and its title – the pandemic has also opened an unprecedented path for immunization itself. To begin with, in a metaphorical sense: the most recent studies of the body's immune system have abandoned the time-worn defensive image of invading germs. This is not to say that it has faded away: the defense function is more critical than ever in combatting the virus. But it must be placed in a wider and more complex biological scenario, in which the immune system is not so much a rigid barrier that protects individual identity as a dialectical filter vis-à-vis the external environment, which inhabits it from the beginning. In the continual lexical transit between the political and the biological, the biological can stop being the natural cage of the political and become instead its symbolic referent – in other words, the immune system's opening to otherness can symbolize political systems' opening to the other. Our immune system shows better than anything how we can and must welcome the external inside ourselves, making our bodies into a place of continual exchange and passage between the inside and the outside.

But this metaphorical allusion, drawn from the immune paradigm, has been replaced recently by another, which is explicitly political. I am referring to the relationship between immunity and community. We know that they are opposites, both logically and etymologically. But this does not preclude their mutual co-belonging. In reality, one cannot exist without the other. Up until now, though, throughout modern history at least, immunization has cut through community, separating it into inversely proportional zones: the protection, or privilege, of one part of humanity has always been countered by the extreme vulnerability and exposure of another. Even in medicine, a process of universal immunization, intended for the whole world, has never been conceived of, or even imagined. For the first time in history, this is exactly what is being proposed today: vaccination for the entire human race. No one is more aware than me of the historical, political, and economic difficulties that this project presents, not to mention the tensions, disagreements, and conflicts it is bound to provoke. While the production and the distribution of the vaccine erase certain geopolitical boundaries, they carve out others, perhaps even deeper ones, between those who possess the means of production and those who have little chance of acquiring them. We shall see how this plays out, how effectively political forces are able to assert their liberating demands – if they still have any – against narrower but no less tenacious established interests. The fact remains, however, that this demand for universal immunization arises not only from individuals but also from governments and political forces. For the first time, I repeat, we glimpse the emergence – at least in some people's intentions – of a possible overlap of community and immunity that could well receive the paradoxical name of "common immunity."

1

Contaminations

1

My research on this topic began with the assumption that "community" and "immunity" are so tightly bound together that they can never be thought of separately. Although I wrote individual books on each concept – titled respectively *Communitas*[1] and *Immunitas*[2] – I approached them from the perspective of their original relationship. In reality, even to speak of a "relationship" may be reductive of a more intrinsic connection, which points instead to a kind of contradictory copresence. Community and immunity are two sides of a single semantic block, which acquires meaning precisely from their tension. This semantic inextricability is made evident, on the etymological plane as well, by their shared lemma – the Latin polysemous noun *munus*, with its meanings "obligation," "burden," and "duty," but also "gift." From it derive both *communitas* and *immunitas* – the former directly and affirmatively, the latter in a negative or privative form. While members of a *communitas* – which, in its broadest application, embraces all human beings – share a donative obligation toward others, those who declare themselves, or are declared, *immunes* ("free from") are exempt from it. Their only relationship with *communitas* is through exemption: as Latin dictionaries tell us, the immune are those who are exempt *a muneribus* – from the obligations (*munera*) that others take on. But, rather than focusing on exemption from *munus* in order to grasp the most distinctive meaning of *immunitas*, we do better to look at the fundamental contrast between it and *communitas*: according to the same dictionaries, he who does not perform the offices that *omnibus communia sunt* – "are common to everyone" – is said to be immune. So, more than being free from the burden of *munus*, immune signifies *not* being common: someone who is immune breaks the donative circuit implicit in *communitas*, relating to it as a negative relates to a positive. *Immunitas* is expressed only in relation to that which it negates or from which it removes itself. If there were no pre-existing, common *munus* to honor – no collective commitment to fulfil – there would be no possibility of exoneration either. To place oneself in a situation of distinction or privilege, one must necessarily presuppose a general condition from which to detach oneself. If there were no common bond to be released from, the very meaning of immunity would be lost.

When we emphasize immunity's negative character, however, we should not attribute it solely to the fundamental contrast with community but also, as noted earlier, to its negative mode of action. From this point of view, alongside the juridical meaning of exemption from a particular law, we must also turn to the biomedical sense of the word, namely protection from an infectious disease. As we know, in the phenomenon of natural or acquired immunity, the practice of vaccination involves incorporating a fragment of the illness that we want to protect ourselves from: the presence of the antigen is what activates the biological organism's protective antibodies. Recalling the ambivalent meaning of the ancient *pharmakon*, we might say that the medicine is mixed with the poison, consumed in a dosage compatible with the body's health. Here again we see the productive role of negation, used sustainably to confront a greater negative: death. The western philosophical tradition has invented countless variations of the negative, of which Hegel's dialectic is the best known. But perhaps none has a richer semantic profile than the enigmatic figure of the *katechon*, which is used by Paul the Apostle in his letters and, not surprisingly, reappears with various meanings throughout modern and contemporary political theology. Like the immune process, the *katechon* is the shield, the brake that resists the supreme evil – the apocalypse – not by directly opposing it but, on the contrary, by incorporating and holding it in itself. This explains its intrinsic connection with the immune *dispositif*. Like the *katechon*, the latter, too, has a negative mode of action. Actually it is doubly negative: posited already as the reverse of *communitas*, it cares for the community not directly but by using a portion of the evil from which it seeks to save it. This is how immunity turns out to be inextricably bound to its opposite. It exists only in relation to the community, which it protects and contradicts at the same time.

But this is only the first side of the issue; it must be completed by the other, inverse and complementary side. Just as, logically, there can be no immunity without community, in the same way, historically, there can be no community without immunity. To understand this interdependence, we must return to the original meaning of *communitas* as a reciprocal gift. As a purely donative relationship, it is formed not by subjects united through the same belonging but, on the contrary, by what puts their respective identities at risk. From this point of view, understood in its most universal mode, *communitas* is different from, and actually opposite to, the identity-making communities associated with today's neocommunitarianism. Unlike them, it relates not so much to something owned – a property – as to an expropriation, a lack of what is one's own or "proper." This makes it elusive theoretically – and even more so historically: a community of this sort is incapable of existing, hence the need to relate it to an immune *dispositif* that, by denying an unlimited opening for it, makes it historically possible and recognizable. For this lack of substance, this "nothing in common," to manifest itself in reality, it must be partially filled up by its opposite. This means that, once the concept of *communitas*, in itself undifferentiated, is plunged into historical reality, it always requires some form of immunization that allows it to endure in time. Without an immune system to defend it, no body politic could survive any more than a human body the dangers that threaten it from within and from without.

When Ferdinand Tönnies opposed community to society[3] as ideal types of social groups, in reality he inferred community from society, as its negative form. That kind of community was simply a society conceived of in reverse. In the historical reality, all societies are immunized to a greater or lesser degree. For good reason, the community he described had all the closed and defensive characteristics of immunity. In effect there is no such thing as communities without immune mechanisms; without them they would not survive the test of time. In this sense, far from being a simple opposite, immunization is the destiny or precondition of every community. Whatever one may wish for, historical communities are always determined by boundaries, external and internal: external, to distinguish them from other communities, and internal, to structure their population in groups based on different ranks, power, and wealth. No society, even the most homogeneous, has known absolute parity between its members, which is why immunization is not a subjective option for any body politic but rather a structural given. It cuts through the community along lines of inclusion and exclusion that, by qualifying its members socially and politically, make them different from one another.

For this reason, the copresence of community and immunity is essentially problematic. In essence it contradicts the meaning of each, understood in its purity. The idea that immunization constitutes the historical mode of every community is at odds with the original meaning of community as an undifferentiated opening, pressing it hard against its opposite. To this inevitable antinomy we owe the tension that courses through every community, exposing it to continuous conflict over the ways and forms of its immunization. Immunization takes on different gradations, which distinguish different societies. No society, except a totalitarian one, is ever entirely immunized. Their degree of immunization depends on external events and internal power relations. Politics can also be defined as the activity that regulates – intensifies or mitigates – the immunization processes in various social environments. To be realistic, it must assume that the immune process is inevitable; and it must seek to mitigate it as much as possible. Only by knowing the limit that runs through a community can politics limit that limit still further, thereby preventing the immune *dispositif* from breaking the common bond and drifting toward an autoimmune tendency. There is always a limit point, a threshold, beyond which the immune process, inward- and outward-facing, tends to grow until it disrupts the equilibrium with its own common measure, giving rise to something similar to an autoimmune disease. When viewed from this angle, community and immunity are impossible to conceive of outside the aporetic node that their copresence creates.

2

In the first book I wrote on immunity, which the present one develops, I highlighted the fruitfulness of the immune paradigm in defining biopolitics. It fills in the gap between the words "life" and "politics" that Foucault had left open to some extent – a point emphasized by subsequent interpreters. When it comes to the oscillation between a hypernegative conception, in which power ravages life, and another, markedly affirmative, in which life absorbs power into its own ontological flow, the immunization paradigm offers the advantage of creating a connection capable of integrating them into a single semantic block. What makes this possible is a non-absolute characterization of the negative. In "immunitary" logic, the negative is not the oppressive or exclusionary force that power exerts over life, as much as the way in which life survives, taking distance from its own internal energy, which could be disintegrative. When we define immunity as a negative protection of life, we mean that immunity does not protect life directly – in an immediate, frontal fashion – but by subjecting it to a constraint that diminishes its vital potency, channeling that power within certain borders.

That said, we can also look at the matter by flipping the coin to the other side. Just as the immune paradigm permits a more adequate definition of biopolitics than Foucault's paradigm, biopolitics, too, has a bearing on how the immune paradigm is interpreted.[4] What is in question here is not the two constitutive poles of biopolitics but rather the two sides of immunity: the legal–political and the biomedical. The former, as we have seen, regards the exemption of certain individual or collective subjects from common duties, while the latter concerns someone's natural or induced protection from an infectious disease. From our point of observation, the two elements seem to coexist naturally within the concept of immunity. Whether we refer to one or the other of its meanings depends on the context of one's discussion. But what looks like natural coexistence to our contemporary gaze is in reality the product of a long history, in which the two meanings of the word followed each other in time and were integrated into a single lemma, only much later. What appears to us as synchrony, almost as coexistence, is the optical effect of a clear-cut chronological distance: the legal–political side of immunity precedes the biomedical side by at least two thousand years.[5] Although references to biological immunity appear quite early in texts – for example in Lucan's *Pharsalia*, on the occasion of describing an African tribe's resistance to snake venom – the legal–political meaning becomes specialized long before the biomedical one and influences it quite markedly. When biological immunity is represented as a form of defense, or even counterattack, of a given body against foreign invaders – as microbes and virus germs are defined – a political–military jargon is being introduced into the language of medicine.[6] Similarly, the definition of the immunological "self" as a solid entity, differentiated from other living bodies and the surrounding environment, transcribes into medical language the idea of modern individualism. The entire lexicon with which the science of immunology was born at the end of the nineteenth century is drawn almost entirely from the language of politics. It was not Hobbes and Locke – with their respective ideas of protecting life and personal identity – who, in an anticipatory fashion, adopted the language of immunology, which did not exist in their time. It happened the other way round: it was rather immunology that absorbed from these authors the concept of a self that defends itself from external attacks and of a personal entity endowed with a memory capable of preserving its identity over time. On the side of philosophical and political models, one can hardly underestimate the importance of this semantic transfer for a medical science destined to assume greater importance over time. But the striking thing is the lack of questioning, on the side of immunological science, about the effects of this metaphorical incorporation. For more than half a century, and to some extent still today, almost no commentator seems to be aware of the performative effects of this lexical slippage. A quick look through the most widely read immunology textbooks suffices for us to see this blind spot behind the definitions.[7] Thinking of the immune system as a battery of soldiers engaged in no-holds-barred combat against external invaders halted immunological science in an immature phase, which it has managed to surpass only in recent decades, not without difficulties and setbacks.

It is true, as we will see in more detail, that this was not a one-way direction, from politics to biology, since the biological side of immunity reacted to the political side in reverse, influencing it in its turn. To recall the most notorious and extreme example, consider how the Nazis used the jargon of infectology against the Jewish people – depicting them as germs, bacteria, and viruses to be exterminated. And they were exterminated, in fact. Over the course of modern history, the performative power of the metaphor acted in both directions – from politics to biology and from biology to politics. But, in terms of genealogy, there remains an almost two-thousand-year distance that separates the two meanings of the concept of immunity. For more than two thousand years, that is, until the late nineteenth century, the only meaning of immunity in use was the legal–political one, of safe conduct conferred on certain subjects who were exempt from current laws. This sense of the word was so prevalent that it remained almost unchanged for millennia. Whatever name it took, a kind of legal immunity was in practice as far back as the earliest Mediterranean civilizations, in a form not that different from what the diplomatic corps still enjoys today in international law. Politicians, heads of state, and members of parliament are also still protected from the general justice system through various kinds of immunity.[8] As for ecclesiastical immunity, which the very existence of the Vatican state confirms, its age-old role has never been challenged.

In chronological perspective, to see when the concept of legal immunity became established, we must go back to the ancient republic of Rome. In the legal system it developed – which no civilization, past and present, rivals in complexity and power of transmission – *immunitas* designated the particular status of certain segments of the population, or even towns, vis-à-vis the general rules.[9] We should not lose sight of the literally antinomic character – simultaneously *intra legem* (within the law) and *extra legem* (outside the law) – of the legal immunity *dispositif*. It is an exemption from the law that the law itself established. When the law declares someone to be immune, it places that individual in a space outside its circle, yet without giving up on legally defining his or her prerogatives. He or she is legally legitimized to overstep the law. Indeed, nothing validates a rule in its generality more than an exemption from it – this is exactly how every exception proves the rule that it breaks. The moment the biological meaning of immunity took its place alongside the legal one, absorbing the political–military jargon, it incorporated the same aporetic structure. When shielding certain individuals from the risk of infection, medical immunization, too, places them in a zone of exception that in some way confirms, negatively, the danger to which everyone else is still exposed – unless the entire community is immunized. Of course, this is not a statutory law but rather a law of nature. It should not be forgotten, however, that the law of nature forms an integral part of a prominent tradition of modern law: *ius naturale*. In this respect, too, then, biology absorbs an element from jurisprudence, in a sort of double compound that is at once ontological and epistemological. Thus the law is made into biological material and biological material is made into a law that can be transgressed without being violated.

The shift in the concept of immunity from one sense to the other obviously brought several consequences with it: for example, what is defined as "biopolitics" is at the same time a presupposition and an effect. In historical terms, the precondition for the shift from law to biology was the rise of social medicine. In its turn, the politicization of medicine in the twentieth century was the consequence of the fact that the concept of immunity shifted onto the biological terrain. Only then did a sort of hybrid take form, which, paraphrasing Clausewitz, made medicine the continuation of politics by other means. Similarly, it can be argued that, just as for Carl Schmitt all modern political concepts have a theological origin, all biomedical concepts – at least the immunological ones – have a political origin. The only difference is that the locus where this semantic transfer occurred was not a branch of knowledge but the bodies of individuals and populations. The body became the battleground between the clashing forces of health and illness, but also between rules and exceptions. From this point of view, we might say that the modern shift from the political to the biological is in keeping with the metaphor that compares the body politic to the human body, which goes much further back in the philosophical tradition. This is how politics and biology, like history and nature, continually exchange their semantic commutators. Something that once appeared natural becomes historical, while something that is historical ends up becoming naturalized. Thus, if on the one hand germs were identified with human armies that attack the living body, in the midtwentieth century humans would be likened to germs that should be eradicated without trace.

3

When we say that legal immunity came far before biological immunity, we are referring to conceptual paradigms, of course, not to the historical reality. As long as human beings have lived, they have always had an immune system, without which they would not have been able to survive. This has not been enough to reduce the very high mortality rate that was due to major epidemic diseases – smallpox, influenza, tuberculosis, malaria, plague, measles, cholera, and others – which have literally decimated the world's population. To go back as far as possible, even the disappearance of *Homo neanderthalensis* seems to have been the result of a smallpox epidemic. It is estimated that, in Europe alone, this disease killed half a million people a year for at least eighteen centuries. Clearly these natural traumas had determinative effects on political-historical events. From the plague of Athens to the twentieth-century Spanish flu, endemic diseases have played a more decisive role in human history than one might imagine.[10] World War II did not have the catastrophic consequences of the previous world war because soldiers on both sides were largely vaccinated.

Awareness of both the sociopolitical importance of epidemic diseases and the immunization processes that have been used to tackle them at various times remains low. Consequently, while the role that General Winter played in forcing Napoleon's troops to retreat during the Russian campaign of 1812 is well known, the equally important role of "General Typhus" is less so. In his popular book *Guns, Germs, and Steel*, Jared Diamond attempts to fill this hermeneutic lacuna by calling attention to the extraordinary importance of immunity in political history. Its strategic weight in interhuman conflicts has been fundamental. As he writes, an infectious disease transmitted by relatively immune invaders to indigenous peoples who lacked immune defenses has been "one of the key factors in world history."[11] Indeed, germs brought by Europeans to America were much more effective at conquering it than weapons were: they exterminated up to 90 percent of the local population. This happened wherever the Europeans arrived: in Australia, South Africa, and all the way to the islands of Fiji, Hawaii, and Tonga. But what happened in America is particularly striking, because of the staggering disproportion between a tiny number of conquistadores and the overwhelming preponderance of the subjugated peoples. In a very short period in 1531, with only 168 men, Francisco Pizarro took possession of the vast Incan Empire, where smallpox, which had arrived a few years earlier, had already killed the emperor and his heir to the throne. Similarly, the 8 million inhabitants of Hispaniola disappeared almost entirely in a matter of forty years, once they encountered the European invaders. The teeming American Indian population that used to live in the Mississippi valley was also largely wiped out by the epidemic, even before Hernando de Soto arrived there.[12]

But the most staggering conquest via epidemic remains that of the Aztec Empire: although populated by 20 million inhabitants, it was taken by a few hundred men led by Hernán Cortés.[13] Smallpox – brought to Mexico in 1520 by a slave from the Spanish colony of Cuba – was certainly not the only cause of the Aztec collapse. Military supe-riority, naval technology, and strategic skill contributed significantly to the Spanish victory. But without small-pox, which cut down more than half of Montezuma's soldiers, it is unlikely that the empire would have crum-bled. According to accounts of the time, what most struck the Aztecs, chipping away at their morale more than the military defense, was the invaders' apparent invulnerabil-ity to the disease that was emptying their ranks. Simply put, the war was won by the Spaniards' immunity to the virus that they had transported to America on their ships. Persuaded by an ancient prophecy that predicted the feathered serpent god Quetzalcoatl would return that year, and seeming to recognize the god's features in Cortés, Montezuma became convinced that ruin was inevitable and delivered himself to his enemies. When even his brother and successor Cuitláhuac died of smallpox, the game was over: the Spaniards easily had the better of the surviving native people. Their immunity, it could be said, defeated the Aztec community, which was exposed naturally to the contagion.

But why did the Spaniards possess the immunity that the Aztecs lacked? What makes some peoples less predis-posed than others to become ill from certain infectious diseases? Why are some populations immune when others are not? Diamond's answer points to three factors that put the Native Americans at an immunological disad-vantage with respect to the European invaders. First of all, New World societies were younger than those of the Old World; hence they would have had fewer opportuni-ties to come into contact with viruses that the Europeans had experienced for a long time. Second, the American populations, distributed as they were over a larger area – from the Andes to Central America and the Mississippi Valley – had never come into contact with one another; but this occurred frequently in Eurasia. Finally, Native Americans knew far fewer domesticated animals than the livestock that Europeans had lived with for a very long time. These animals had been transmitting their viruses to Europeans over the course of generations and had thus immunized them from subsequent contaminations. All this reduced the circulation of viral agents on the American continent and stopped the formation of an immunological memory that the Europeans had already acquired. The last factor turns out to be the most important. The worst killers of humanity are diseases that transmigrate across species, jumping from animal to human bodies. For this reason – the habitual coexistence of domesticated animals – agricultural societies are more exposed to the spread of viruses. Of course, this is predicated on numbers of individuals large enough to allow the viruses to circulate and replicate. It is estimated that, in a community of fewer than 5,000 individuals, a virus tends to die out sooner or later, for lack of hosts able to transmit it.

According to Jean Ruffié,[14] a historian of epidemics, there is another reason that explains Native Americans' weak immune response by comparison with that of Europeans: their monomorphism, or at least weak polymorphism, which is due more to selective pressures than to chance. It is thought that monomorphism originated with the first migrations into the New World of peoples who arrived in four waves from Siberia across the frozen Bering Strait. Evidence for this provenance comes from both common genetic elements and linguistic affinities between the inhabitants of Upper Asia and those of North America. We know that monomorphism – low variability in the cluster of genes that make up the major histocompatibility complex of certain ethnic groups – limits the immune response to infectious agents. This is because polymorphism produces a high level of antigens capable of generating antibodies, whereas monomorphism, on the contrary, is deficient in this respect. True, even in populations with a certain degree of polymorphism some individuals do not possess the necessary molecules to form a substantial group of antigens; but this defect is compensated for by the presence of diverse individuals, who have them in abundance. This does not happen by default in monomorphism, because the individuals' genetic variety is quite limited. This immune fragility caused by monomorphism is precisely what exposed the American Indians to viral infection. Obviously, an endogenous factor is not enough to trigger a demographic catastrophe like the one that occurred in Central and North America unless it is associated with an exogenous factor, namely the arrival of an infection brought in by external invaders. But, once arrived, the contagion spreads all the more easily as the immune system of local populations is less resistant, and they are left defenseless against a double enemy that is both military and epidemic. This is why monomorphism, or limited polymorphism, was simultaneously the cause and the effect of the demographic collapse. It was the cause because it weakened the host population to external viruses. It was the effect because the military decimation of the defeated population reduced genetic variety even further.

The Spanish conquest adds cultural and symbolic factors to this vicious circle. Their arrival appeared to the American Indians not as a completely new event but as a replica of a long-feared one: a repeat of the first invasion of the Asian populations. When Aztecs, Mayans, and Incas saw white, bearded men arriving from the sea, whose images their ancestors had deposited in their memory, they likened them to divinities that it would have been useless to resist and therefore delivered themselves into their hands. The indigenous peoples' muted response in the face of their executioners, a font of great surprise to European observers, stemmed from a supernatural interpretation of historical events. A purely historical set of events appeared to them as inexorable destiny. What transpired from the conjunction of political-historical phenomena – the Spaniards' strategic and military superiority – and natural givens – the immune fragility of peoples with weak polymorphism – laid the conditions for one of the most horrifying hecatombs in human history.

4

The politicization of medicine – beginning in Europe in the early eighteenth century – is central to Foucault's work. It would be inaccurate to say that he uses the immune paradigm to interpret it. Indeed, his lack of reference to the immune paradigm prevents him from fully developing the concept of biopolitics. Nevertheless, even though Foucault does not talk explicitly about it, immunization runs across his entire reconstruction of the history of European medicine. This is clear from the decisive role in redefining the medical gaze that he assigns to the fight against epidemics. *The Birth of the Clinic* already identifies this fight as the turning point that leads from the old medicine of classes, still built on the botanical model, to a clinic guided by historically determined, collective phenomena. An epidemic is now something that attacks a large number of people over a given period and through the same characteristics – "a sort of over-all singularity, an individual with many similar heads, whose features are manifested only once in time and space."[15] Even if person-to-person transmission of the infection was not viewed as the primary cause of an epidemic – identified instead with some miasma supposed to circulate in the air – it required widespread surveillance, which went beyond the medical regime and involved the political and administrative sphere.

This produced an initial politicization of medicine, which had a corresponding response at the institutional level. After founding the Royal Academy of Medicine, still at the height of the *ancien régime*, the French government established at Versailles a commission responsible for dealing with epidemic phenomena and epizootic diseases. It had three roles: investigation, elaboration, and prescription. A double system of checks and controls was set up; at first it targeted the physicians themselves, whose training was taken away from academic bodies and assigned to centralized organizations under direct governmental responsibility, and then was extended to the entire population via the gathering of statistics and a systematic observation of cases. A further shift toward the political came about during the Revolution, when responsibility for pathological phenomena was assigned to society, under the banner of national interest. Attention to infectious diseases and to immune measures for containing them was heightened through this initiative. The primary task of the *cour de salubrité* ("health court") established in Paris was to reconstruct the chain of infection through a network formed by the intersection of cases in a defined territorial space. This did not mean ignoring the individual aspect of the disease but placing it in a wider circle of a social nature. It is as if the medical gaze split into two overlapping roles, one personal, the other collective. At work in this conception was the revolutionary myth of a fight against disease that paralleled the fight against social privileges, almost as if medicine should take over from the church a task that was also salvific. Just as the church ministered to souls, medicine took charge of the citizens' bodies, joined together in the sacred body of the nation. The outcome was intensely political: "The first task of the doctor is therefore political: the struggle against disease must begin with a war against bad government. Man will be totally and definitively cured only if he is first liberated."[16]

In *The Birth of the Clinic*, the immune question arises from Foucault's analysis of the epidemic; in his lectures on social medicine given in Rio de Janeiro, it takes center stage. He starts by deconstructing a cliché that opposes modern medicine, privately oriented, to the collectively oriented medicine practiced in medieval times. That is not how things were in reality. Capitalism socialized its object – the bodies of its workers, that is – from the very beginning, with the aim of increasing the collective labor force. This dynamic is an integral part of the biopolitical turn, which Foucault theorized in his courses at the Collège de France during the same years: "For capitalist society, it was biopolitics, the biological, the somatic, the corporeal, that mattered more than anything else. The body is a biopolitical reality; medicine a biopolitical strategy."[17] In the society of late modernity, this politicization process developed beyond any expectation. Medicine acted well beyond its traditional frontiers, encroaching upon a much more extensive territory, to the point of filling in all the gaps between areas. As Foucault observes in the first of his two Rio lectures,

> What is diabolical about the present situation is that whenever we want to refer to a realm outside medicine we find that it has already been medicalized. And when one wishes to object to medicine's deficiencies, its drawbacks and its harmful effects, this is done in the name of a more complete, more refined and widespread medical knowledge.[18]

Of course, this recent outcome is but the last stretch in a long process, whose first stages took place in Prussia, France, and England. The first is represented by medicine in the German state. Early in the sixteenth and seventeenth centuries, in France and England the authorities began to measure the power of the population through birth and death rate surveys, censuses, and health indexes, although this information gathering never turned into direct interventions to protect and improve public health, as it did in Germany with the institution of a *medizinische Polizei* or *Polizei der Medizin* ("medical police"). As is well known, the eighteenth-century concept of "police" has a much broader semantic range than the current one. At that time, it signified the economic and military but also biological government of the population for the purpose of reinforcing the state. To achieve such an end, a normalization of medical knowledge took place over time, aimed at bringing it under government control. Before he was a technician of healing, the German doctor was a state functionary who administered health, treated like any other government branch. In line with the trends of cameralism and mercantilism, an increasingly bureaucratic medicine protected the state's collective force in the bodies of individuals. In this correspondence between medicine, law, and politics we can already recognize the two sides of the immunization process: protection from endemic diseases is inseparable from protection from the state apparatus, through a continual reversibility between biological security and social security.

The second step in the politicization of medical knowledge, and one that was even more deeply intrinsic to immunitary logic, is represented by urban medicine in France. Urban medicine was fueled by a growing fear of citizen assemblies, a fear with both biological and social roots. For example, the late eighteenth-century philosopher Pierre Jean Gioerge Cabanis argued that "whenever men came together their morals changed for the worse; whenever they came together in closed places their morals and their health deteriorated."[19] In the face of the expansion of new urban masses, a sort of politico-sanitary anxiety rippled through the middle classes. Confronted by these new epidemic risks, they resorted, albeit in a more sophisticated form, to the old medieval quarantine – the most primitive, but also the most effective immune *dispositif* ever. The quarantine strategy has the simplicity of mathematical division: each family in a single house and, when possible, each person in a single room. In conformity with a *quadrillage* system that reproduced an ancient immune practice, the city was rigidly divided into districts and neighborhoods. This is the individualizing plague model, as opposed to the exclusionary leprosy model. According to a paradox still recurrent today, society as a whole can be saved only by isolating each individual it comprises. Areas of communal use – cemeteries, slaughterhouses, washhouses – were moved to locations outside the city walls. Like the living, the dead, too, were dug up from their common grave and buried in individual coffins, for health and hygiene reasons much more than for religious ones. Public hygiene was the lynchpin of immune medicine, at least before vaccination. The transition from the idea of healthiness to that of hygiene marked a change of intensity as well as of scale. The relationship between environment and organism – later picked up in different ways by Cuvier and Lamarck – stood at the crossroads between the natural sciences and urban medicine. What mattered was to control the circulation of people and things and to channel them along separate paths. The new, modern city was born of this immunitary need: streets were widened, buildings were ventilated, and rivers were embanked. The bigger the collective space grew, the more it was distributed into separate spheres.

In the third phase, represented by English labor force medicine, the immunitary knots are tied even tighter. Perception of the subordinate classes' poverty changed with the development of capitalism, exacerbating the ruling classes' anxieties. Earlier, the poor were included in the circle of citizenship in order to perform socially useful jobs, such as delivering the mail, transporting water, taking away the garbage; now they begin to be perceived as a social aggregate that one should protect and be protected from at the same time. The Poor Law, which was in effect at the time of the cholera epidemic that originated in Paris in 1832 and spread across Europe, had a significance that was both sanitary and political. It expressed on the one hand solidarity with the "needy," in conformity with an ancient charitable model, and on the other a need for social control in the form of a rigidly selective and exclusionary cordon of immunity.

> In this way, an officially sanctioned sanitary cordon between the rich and the poor was set in place within the cities. To that end, the latter were offered the possibility of receiving free or low-cost treatment. Thus, the wealthy freed themselves of the risk of being victims of epidemic phenomena issuing from the disadvantaged classes.[20]

In the late nineteenth century, when the Health Service would take over from the Poor Law, rationalizing it through science, the security paradigm extended potentially to the entire population, through immune prevention measures applied to people, objects, and environments – without undermining the economic and biological dominance of the wealthy classes, of course, and even bolstering it. The emerging system took the form of three overlapping but not coinciding layers: a welfare medicine for the poorest; an administrative medicine for matters concerning the whole population; and a private medicine benefiting the wealthiest.

5

The decisive moment for the immune paradigm – as far as it concerned state, regional, and urban health policies – came with the discovery and spread of vaccination in the first half of the nineteenth century. As often happens in the history of medicine, practical experimentation preceded theoretical developments. Priority in using the "variolation" method of inoculation – the artisanal precursor of real vaccination – was contested by countries whose claims were more geopolitical than medical in tone.[21] The Jesuit priest Père d'Entrecolles located the first inoculation experiments in tenth-century China. A few centuries later, similar practices spread throughout the Ottoman Empire, as reported by the British ambassador to Constantinople, Lady Mary Wortley Montagu, to whom we owe one of the first attempts to export variolization to England. During the same period, two Greek physicians in Padua, Emmanuel Timoni and Jacob Phylarini, disseminated the use of variolation, making it public in a letter to the Royal Society of London. When smallpox arrived in Boston in the early 1700s, Cotton Mather, a distinguished local physician, put out a patent on variolation in Massachusetts. His book, *Angel of Bethesda*[22] – one of the first medical texts produced in colonial America – contains a chapter called "Variola Triumphata, or the Small-Pox Encountred" in which he argues that immunity to smallpox can be achieved by injecting viral material drawn from patients who suffer from a mild form of the same disease. There was an idea, halfway between popular belief and empirical fact, that circulated for some time – namely that someone who has recovered from an illness cannot reproduce it. This led people to infect themselves on purpose, using the pus of a sick person, which almost always ended in death. The method risked not only failing to achieve immunization but also spreading the infection further.

In this murky picture, in which magical hypotheses alternated with therapeutic prescriptions, the first experiment capable of producing real curative effects was conducted at the end of the century by the English country doctor Edward Jenner, from Berkeley in Gloucestershire. Probably influenced by his teacher John Hunter – who believed that it was impossible for the same illness to recur in a patient – he began to study the phenomenon systematically in 1788, setting the stage for immunological studies. We know the event that proved to be decisive, despite being unplanned. Jenner extracted purulent matter from a pustule of smallpox transmitted to a milkmaid from cows; he injected it into an eight-year-old boy, then followed it with another inoculation, this time from a man sick with smallpox, thus demonstrating that the boy had become immune. From then on, the term "vaccine" – derived from the Latin *vacca*, "cow" – was extended to all kinds of substances with the power to stop an infectious disease. At this point the original practice of person-to-person variolation, which had highly problematic effects in terms of risk and inefficiency, was replaced by vaccination, which proved to be safe and effective. Despite Jenner's discovery, the new procedure encountered several difficulties – even from the Royal Society, which refused to legitimize it, judging its principles to be revolutionary and its results unreliable. To secure his copyright over the technique, Jenner then self-published a book called *An Inquiry into the Causes and Effects of the* variolae vaccinae, *a Disease Known by the Name of Cow Pox*, in which the word "virus" was used for the first time.[23] From that moment on, his theory – perhaps better described as a practice – was adopted rapidly all over Europe, quickly "Jennerized," and then exported to the colonies to combat the horrible epidemics often imported by the European colonizers themselves. In the span of a few years, a hundred thousand people were vaccinated in Europe, while Napoleon had his son vaccinated in 1805 and then extended mandatory vaccination to the entire French population. In a series of acts issued between 1840 and 1871, English legislation also made vaccination mandatory, marking a point of no return in containment strategies for infectious diseases. By comparison, vaccination appeared to be the only immune strategy able to combat viruses with equal ammunition. It was a decisive shift. With the spread of vaccines, for the first time the ancient but never abandoned procedure of quarantine became a last resort, to be implemented only in the absence of a vaccine.

These are the historical steps that marked the genesis and then the extraordinary success of Jenner's discovery. However, the question of its fundamental meaning in relation to the immune paradigm remains to be considered. Not only did it make it more powerful, placing it front and center in the fight against humanity's most frightening natural enemies; it signaled an even tighter bond between the two categories of *immunitas* and *communitas*, antinomically incorporating one into the other. Certainly, immunizing someone through a vaccine means isolating that person from those who are not vaccinated – hence from the rest of the community, assuming of course that not everyone can be vaccinated, a condition that never failed to be true. But, from another point of view, the vaccine, which was obtained initially from other sick people and later, in Jenner's famous experiment, from animals, represents a breach of barriers not only between individuals but also between species. Obviously, today's vaccination methods have evolved enormously by comparison with those primitive ones, thanks to biological technologies that preserve almost nothing of Jenner's first experiments. Still, something connected to them remains discernible, so to speak, in the terminology used today to define certain vaccination practices or effects. When we talk, as we did even recently, of *herd immunity*, are we not conjuring up the species of animal from which the name "vaccination" derives?

Even more, herd immunity, also defined as "common immunity," is located on the borderline between immunity and community, bringing one near to the other. The explicit contiguity between humans and animals, a proximity that evokes the "pastoral government" in which Foucault recognized the birth of modern biopolitics, translates the intention to protect not only the vaccinated but, through them, the entire community. This does not alter the fact that the option of herd immunity announced by some governments carries with it a thanatopolitical residue that appears to flip the biopolitical paradigm into its deadly reverse. This is what happens when herd immunity, once it has not been achieved by means of vaccination, seeks to take its place, aiming for natural instead of vaccine-based immunization. This method is based on the possibility that, when immunization has reached a sizable percentage of the population through widespread contamination, the virus will be brought to a halt, because it has nowhere left to circulate. The thanatopolitical assumption behind this strategy, however, is that, since not everyone can be vaccinated, we can abandon the most vulnerable to the virus in order to avoid an economically damaging total closure. Thus, far from integrating into *communitas* – into the general interest, that is – *immunitas* comes to constitute its starkest opposite: in the most sinister fashion, it brings into reality Foucault's pronouncement that contemporary biopolitics allows people to live by abandoning those who remain outside the circle of economic reproduction, by letting them die. The fact that, sometimes after a rapid about-face, no European government ended up taking this logic to its extremes during the current pandemic does not mean that a solution of this kind was not put forward or that under different circumstances it will not be proposed again.

This is why the importance of the vaccination issue extends beyond healthcare into politics – and for a double reason. The choice of who will be vaccinated – for extending vaccination to everyone was never considered possible until now – has always constituted a political battleground, not only for getting the vaccine but also for avoiding it. In the lecture on social medicine cited earlier, Foucault recalls that in the mid-1800s England, when vaccination was made compulsory for the disadvantaged classes in order to protect the well-to-do, it provoked popular insurrections from dissident movements that sought to assert, paradoxically, "the right to life, the right to get sick, to care for oneself and to die in the manner one wished."[24] What are we to make of these protests that, in some ways and in completely different contexts, have continued to our day? How are we to interpret this "political struggle against politically authoritarian medicalization, the socialization of medicine, the medical control that presses mainly on the poor population"?[25] In a chapter of *Immunitary Life* that deals with the biopolitics of vaccination,[26] Nik Brown interprets these battles against compulsory vaccination as a class struggle between elites and the working class. The tightening of sanctions against those who rebelled against vaccinations in the Victorian era was a response not so much to a sanitary concern as to a need for social control. Through increasingly tougher regulations, the capitalism of that time demanded ownership over workers' bodies. In response, resistance to being vaccinated, often associated with the fight for universal suffrage, was a symbolically relevant rejection of subordinate status from a class that was perpetually exposed to exploitation. In the early twentieth century, when conscientious objection gained acceptance in the face of what appeared to shape itself as sanitary dictatorship, it seemed a significant political conquest. In this case the logic of immunization, aimed at defending the community, encountered the reluctance of one of its segments to subject itself to the impositions of the other.

6

While Jenner's experimental vaccination was the precursor to medical immunization, its first implementation is generally attributed to Pasteur. The French physician added to earlier immune practices by providing a theoretical perspective. What in Jenner remained at the level of empirical experimentation, only generalizable after the fact, in Pasteur became a law of biology: once isolated in a laboratory, if processed in a certain way, the bacterium loses its virulence, until it becomes harmless. He realized that, when bacteria are artificially stimulated, their strength eventually diminishes, until it fades out altogether. From that moment on, the introduction of new bacteria did not produce any further growth. He deduced from this phenomenon that, once interrupted, bacterial growth would no longer reproduce itself. In short, after a natural infection or an infection induced through the inoculation of inactivated organisms, the body would not develop the illness again, thus remaining effectively immunized from it. This effect applied, with slight differences, to cholera, anthrax, rabies, and all other types of infectious diseases. The fact that any pathogenic virus could sooner or later weaken was something that humans had always experienced, the moment a given epidemic began to recede. But what had been considered a natural phenomenon became at that point artificially producible, thanks to a particular technique to which Pasteur seemed to possess the keys, in a form that seemed astonishing to his contemporaries; hence the exceptional prestige that soon surrounded his public figure – and the copious funding lavished on his frenetic research activities. People went so far as to say that before him there had been no real medicine, just uncertain and ineffective practices.[27]

But can it really be argued that Pasteur inaugurated the history of immunological science? The answer is not a foregone conclusion. First of all, only rarely does Pasteur use the term "immunity." And even when he does, it refers to a thwarted negative effect more than to a positive activity. Thus, rather than immunization, he speaks of an organism's "refractoriness" to becoming ill, or even of "non-recidivism" – that is, an inability to contract the same disease twice. Even so, the fact alone that the word "recidivism" has legal origins brings us back to the intersection between law and medicine that, as we have seen, characterizes immune semantics. Are these considerations sufficient to make Pasteur the legendary initiator of immunology, as is claimed by a narrative not without hagiographic traits? Certainly, the large-scale use of vaccination amounts to a practice of widespread immunization, although in the case of rabies – the disease of his choice, perhaps because of the spectacular drama of its manifestations – the vaccine is not inoculated preventively, but only in patients who are already infected. This is more of a vaccine therapy, then, than an immunization practice. All in all, before a certain date – up to the 1880s – Pasteur appears more like Jenner's brilliant successor than the inventor of a new field of knowledge. As we have said, vaccination grew out of the *ancien régime*'s medical police, which was later adopted by the revolutionary republic and finally legitimized by Napoleon through his large-scale prescription.

The leap toward an immunitary regime came with the creation of the Pasteur Institute and the propagation of its laboratories, first across France and then overseas, thanks to the invention of what was called "tropical medicine." What rightly deserves the name of "pasteurism" developed at that time as a practice allied with medical sanitization and geopolitical expansion. Bruno Latour has studied the phenomenon in all its implications, at once prophylactic and ideological. Up to a certain point in time, bacteriology was considered a secondary aspect of social hygiene, which was focused on the spaces of the city and, more generally, on air, water, and land. Along with these, at another level, were the states of the body: constitutions, humors, and infections. But what was missing from the social hygiene vision was an element that united the two levels by migrating from the outside to the inside. This element – the "pathogenic agent" – was the microbe, on which Pasteur fixed his sharp gaze. Its presence radically changed medical protocols, but also the image of the entire society. Society was no longer reducible to interpersonal ties, since it now included in its midst horribly noxious inhabitants that were nevertheless invisible. They posed a threat to individual bodies but also, above all perhaps, to the social body as a whole, now attacked by obscure forces that needed to be brought to light, tamed, and, finally, used against themselves. To accomplish this aim – in the never-ending battle between bacteria and vaccines – the commitment of individual doctors was not enough. It required a veritable army in the field, hierarchically organized, with the capability of attacking the enemy and routing it.

Hence a headquarters was created: the Pasteur Institute. It was followed by laboratories all over France, tasked with selecting and cultivating the bacteria, while periodical publications, the *Annales*, developed a two-pronged strategy of defense and attack. Latour describes it as a biopolitical project in grand style, comparable in scope and ambition to Freud's plans for psychoanalysis. Just as the psychoanalyst delved into everyday slips of the tongue in search of mental disturbances, Pasteur searched through the residue of organic life for the parasites that infest the body: "Both [Pasteur and Freud] announced that they were speaking in the name of invisible, rejected, terribly dangerous forces that must be listened to if civilization was not to collapse. Like the psychoanalysts, the Pasteurians set themselves up as exclusive interpreters of populations to which no one else had access."[28]

Like any war, the one launched by the microbe hunters was fought at borders, at the transit points through which viruses pass. The outcome of the match depended entirely on those passageways: "Either the microbe gets through and *all precautions are useless*, or hygienists can stop it getting through and *all other precautions are superfluous.*"[29] Social hygiene was the necessary platform on top of which there arose a new power, at once medical and political – a new politics of medicine. The hybridization between hygienists and Pasteurians reinforced the power of both in a previously nonexistent domain, a realm shared by the parasites and the people who combatted them: "For each parasite, a parasite and a half."[30]

The heart of the struggle – the point where one passes seamlessly from the scientific domain into that of politics and vice versa – was the microbiology laboratory at the École Normale. Ensconced in his laboratory, Pasteur transferred *in vitro* the relation of forces that existed *in vivo*. It was a matter of controlling natural phenomena through artificial methods, overturning the relationship between what is infinitely small and what is infinitely large. With a new biomilitary technology, a handful of people were expected to succeed at dominating the microbial legion that for thousands of years had shown itself to be much stronger than any human being. Just as a parasite of minuscule dimensions can kill an ox or a person billions of times bigger than it, a single generation of humans trained in bacteriological laboratories felt that it could acquire knowledge capable of defeating what had decimated the human species since the dawn of history. The first step in this battle was, paradoxically, to give a name and a face to an enemy that had always lived in the shadows. In this sense, from a certain point of view, Pasteur can be said to have "invented" the microbe. He remodeled what had always existed, distorting its distinguishing features and transferring it into the laboratory. In doing so, he not only made it recognizable, adapting it to his own purposes, but also "discovered" it, not by lifting a veil that covered it but by translating it into medically significant terms. The *Annales* publications are at the forefront of this strategy: a veritable war machine pointed at the variability of microbial virulence. Simply put, science transformed society by doing politics by other means.

There were domestic policies, but also foreign policies. We have already seen that, in the age of the American conquest, smallpox viruses were the most powerful weapon against biologically unprotected Native Americans that the immunized conquistadores had in their possession. Something similar happened during the second colonial wave, activated between the nineteenth and twentieth centuries by the competing European states. This competition was often resolved through military medicine, which in peacetime treated the armed corps and in wartime prevented the soldiers from being ravaged by microbes – microbes that were not always allied with the Whites against the Blacks. In 1802, for example, a French army leaving from Santo Domingo with more than 58,000 men was struck by yellow fever: only 8,000 of them returned to France. A few years later, in 1809, in an expedition to Madagascar against the Hova, the French army suffered an equally devastating massacre. At that point, mass vaccination among soldiers reversed the fortunes of the war, restoring the technological and military superiority that the microbes had canceled out. In a country like France, whose birthrate was in crisis, bacteriological medicine was an irreplaceable ally. The pasteurization of military medicine paved the road for the French colonial venture. From Tangiers to Tunisia and all the way to Saigon, Pasteur became the most influential general in deciding French fortunes; starting in 1908, the *Bulletin de la Société de pathologie exotique* joined the *Annales* in the "foreign policy" of French medicine.

7

But the political importance of immunity methods was not limited to French colonialism. At the end of the nineteenth century, they assumed a decisive role in the struggle between European powers – especially in the bitter clash between France and Germany that culminated in the Franco-Prussian War.[31] This explains the intensely patriotic and nationalistic tones that came to characterize research programs that, in themselves, pertained exclusively to a scientific sphere.

From the very beginning, Pasteur's stance for example, albeit intentionally oriented toward empirical and experimental protocols, displayed a trait that could justifiably be described as political–theological. To identify it, we must dive into the ontogenetic debate of the time, focusing particularly on the theory of spontaneous generation, which was defended primarily by Félix-Archimède Pouchet in *Heterogenesis, or a Treatise of Spontaneous Generation.*[32] Arguing that organic life originates from inanimate matter, this theory broke with the idea of divine creation, thus denying the fundamental doctrine of Christianity; hence the inevitable political–theological outcome this scientific controversy would have. Since a naturally atheistic notion could in principle be used to support anarcho-communist views, Pasteur was quick to take a patriotic stance, insisting that his theory was compatible with Catholic doctrine. In a famous lecture given on April 1, 1864 before a select public that included Alexandre Dumas, George Sand, and Matilde Bonaparte, he vigorously refuted an idea that he considered false and a scandal to the Christian faith. His declaration rang out, not without reason, like a tribute to Napoleon III (Louis Bonaparte), in the hope, soon fulfilled, of obtaining substantial funding for the École Normale laboratory.

After the war, in which his son fought, Pasteur gave a strongly nationalistic and anti-German slant to his position: bacteriological science should serve to treat the "Prussian cancer," that is, to redeem the French. Besides, things were no different on the other side of the Rhine. The same years saw the rising star of Robert Koch, who would become Pasteur's fiercest opponent, both as a scientist and as a popular celebrity. One generation younger than Pasteur, he had begun by working on the anthrax bacterium, discovering it in the blood of infected animals he examined. In Koch's perspective, the pathological process begins when a nutritional competition between organisms of different scales takes place in the body, leading to changes to the previous equilibrium. Like Pasteur, Koch also saw a relationship between infection and bacteria; but he paid closer attention to their specificity. The pathogenic mechanisms that cause multiple diseases such as anthrax, cholera, and typhus turn out to be essentially homologous, it is true. But this does not detract from the peculiar correlation each has with its corresponding bacterium. Koch thus brought more care to the specificity of the microorganisms and to the purity of their *in vitro* isolation than could be found in Pasteur's method, which was judged to be less rigorous. While Pasteur was led to the generalization of a method founded on the variation of bacterial virulence, the German physician limited himself to studying the microorganism's character. What mattered for Koch was not the bacterium's mutation so much as its precise identification. From our current vantage point, their ideas – made largely obsolete by later progress in biotechnology – appear to have more commonalities than divergences. Both scientists worked within the immune paradigm: having identified the pathogenic germs, they use the method of inoculation to prepare therapies of defense against them. But the dominant perception at the time was that their theories were irremediably opposed. This apparent antagonism between therapeutic projects that were in other ways complementary resulted also from an ideological clash with heated nationalistic overtones. If France, badly bruised as it was from a war in which it had lost Alsace-Lorraine, yearned to settle the score, Germany, politically united around that very victory, had every intention of asserting its superiority in the scientific realm as well. The Institute for Infectious Diseases, later named the Robert Koch Institute, was the cutting edge of this imperialist strategy, directed, after the example of its leader, at the French enemy.

This explains the almost epic tone of a bacteriological battle with strong political clout.[33] The fervent anti-German patriotism of the Pasteur Institute was countered with harsh attacks by the German pathologists, who not only denied its therapeutic results but even discredited the institute scientifically. Immunization thus found itself once

again at the biopolitical crossroads of politics and medicine. The process of reciprocal contamination between
these two languages was one of exact, one-to-one correspondence. The political instrumentalization of medicine
was reflected in medicine's tendency to assume a political value. The first report issued by the German Imperial
Health Office – accusing Pasteur of imprecise microbial cultivation – could have easily been titled "Against
Pasteur." From that moment on, the two institutions –
the Pasteur Institute of Paris and the Koch Institute of
Berlin – continued to throw down the gauntlet at each
other for two decades. Victories alternated with defeats
in a no-holds-barred contest flushed with both medicine
and politics. With an incendiary letter, Pasteur handed
back the honorary degree he had received in Bonn from
the Prussian government, provoking indignant reactions
from the German physicians. Although his famous sheep
vaccination experiment at Pouilly le Fort seemed to prove
him right, his adversaries countered by accusing him of
eclecticism, and even of plagiarism. Koch's victory over
his rival in the challenge to identify the cholera bacterium
in the epidemic that broke out in Alexandria prompted
Pasteur to intensify his research on the rabies vaccine – a
discovery that had taken him to the pinnacle of scientific
esteem and personal notoriety. When he had apparently
saved the life of a boy bitten by a rabid dog, he had been
treated as a true hero of the French Pantheon. From then
on, donations to the Pasteur Institute poured in at such a
rate that he was able to set up branches in the Asian colonies. In the meantime, in 1892, Koch had identified the
tuberculosis bacillus. Now a professor at the University
of Berlin, he demanded sanitary inspections across the
entire German territory, thus helping to bolster the central
government's authority. From this point of view, too, he
performed an eminently political role in the Reich as a
physician, receiving the Iron Cross from the emperor and,
in 1905, the Nobel Prize for medicine and physiology.
Scientific discoveries and their political significance are so

intertwined in the immune paradigm during this period that it is especially difficult to disentangle them from each other. As Anne-Marie Moulin writes,

> Hostilities developed between a "French" school and a "German" school – or rather Prussian, embodied by the disciples of Koch. The question of priority between cell and humors got out of proportion. The debate, impassioned, filled every congress, every journal between 1890 and 1910, and fed on the venom around the Alsace-Lorraine problem or of the Jewish question. The war of the scientists was, if not a cause, at least a sign that foreran the conflict of 1914.[34]

Not even Pasteur's death put an end to Franco-German rivalry in immunology. The arrival of the Russian zoopathologist Ilya Ilyich Mechnikov – to whom we owe the first modern concept of biological immunity – opened the second act of a biomedical epic that had yet to grant a definitive victory to either contender. Mechnikov turned his research toward a phenomenon similar to digestion – phagocytosis – and stepped into what had been Pasteur's role, but on a completely new epistemological horizon. His 1901 treatise on immunity[35] seems to have opened a new season in immunological science. Although the existence of white cells had been known for some time, at least from Rudolf Virchow's studies, Mechnikov found that phagocytosis presented an element of active resistance in the organism's fight against infection. What characterizes his work from inception is its opposition to the theory of the humors, which, especially in Germany, drew inspiration from Koch's research. The Russian scientist scored a dazzling victory over his German adversaries at two congresses, held in 1890 in Berlin and in 1894 in Budapest, where he presented the crucial role of phagocytosis. But over the following decades the fortunes of the conflict reversed, and cellular theory was eclipsed by humoral theory. The research inspired by Koch's principles achieved an ascendancy destined to mark immunology for several decades, crowding out cellular theory and, along with it, the "active" notion of immunization. In 1890, Emil Adolf von Behring and Kitasato Shibasaburō discovered that immunity to diphtheria and tetanus was due to antibodies formed in such a way as to exclude any cellular elements from the process. Koch took advantage of the occasion to proclaim the definitive defeat of the phagocytosis theory. The next discovery, by Paul Ehrlich, of the lateral chains that allow antibody receptors to hook onto antigens, put an end to the dispute, leaving cellular theory with an entirely residual role. Although the awarding of the Nobel Prize to Mechnikov[36] and Ehrlich in 1908 attempted to restore a balance between the competing hypotheses, in practice the antibody theory became the only interpretation for understanding immune phenomena, the cellular explanation being now relegated to an outmoded scientific repertoire.

And yet, as often happens in the history of science, this victory did not prove to be definitive either. We will see further on – when transplants, autoimmune diseases, and immune tolerance become major issues – that Mechnikov's perspective was to have its posthumous revenge – not, of course, as it was originally formulated, but by providing the conceptual tools to build the modern idea of immunity. The paradigm's shift from the chemical approach, successful until then, to the biological marked a turning point in a direction that we are still following. Nevertheless, in some ways the political and even military interpretations that dominated immunology at the turn of the twentieth century would never disappear. Even today, when that historical climate appears to be completely behind us, the political connotation of the category of the immune continues to resurface in perpetually new and problematic forms.

2

Autoimmunitarian Democracy

1

For the immune paradigm to unfold in all its ambivalence, inclusive and exclusionary at the same time, we must wait for a second change – the medicalization of politics – that intersects with the first – the politicization of medicine just examined. On this side of the paradigm, entire political systems become immunized, beginning with the system of government that for almost two centuries has taken the ancient name of "democracy." In a book called *La démocratie immunitaire* (*Immunitary Democracy*), Alain Brossat reconstructs this process, connecting it to the dialectic between community and immunity mentioned previously. Starting from a remark by Ernest Renan, according to whom "*Noli me tangere* is the most one can ask for from democracy," he claims that democracy, "understood not only as an institutional regime of politics but, more generally, as a general regime of human life, is fundamentally an *immune system*."[1] Its primary purpose is to ensure that people, things, and opinions are not violated. Even before this guarantee becomes an institutional right, it has the characteristics of a tacit norm, identified with what we call "freedom."

As is typical of the immune paradigm, this is a negative freedom: it does not aim at expanding life but at protecting it from possible risks. Before negative liberty became a stock phrase, it was theorized through contrast to the positive liberty of the ancients, by Benjamin Constant, for whom liberty is "the right to be subjected only to the laws, to be impervious to being arrested, detained, put to death, or maltreated in any way by the arbitrary will of one or more individuals."[2] In other words, it is freedom *from* rather than freedom *of*. What separates the two is a shift from the active concept of participation – implicit in the semantic horizon of *communitas* – to the passive notion of security, understood as exoneration from the constraints and dangers of the common *munus*. This is where modern democracy took its immunitarian turn. Modern democracy is composed of self-protective spheres, invisible but effective, which surround individuals' bodies and actions and make them mutually inviolable. Once immunitarian democracy is encapsulated in the semantics of security, it passes seamlessly and continuously between the originally heterogeneous spheres of politics and medicine, law and biology:

> the immunity paradigm is at work among them [heterogeneous a priori domains], so much so that it creates increasingly important zones of non-differentiation between these different spheres and has the effect that political action, for example, tends to be conceived of under a medical model while, conversely, the problems of medical practice are constantly politicized.[3]

Of course, as has been said, the prerogative of immunity does not belong exclusively to democracy or to modernity. The roots of its juridical meaning go back at least two thousand years – except that, whereas in earlier eras, from the Roman *pater familias* to the absolute monarch, *immunitas* had the character of an exception, in modern democracy it extends, at least in principle, to all individuals. In the *ancien régime*, only the king's body was circumscribed by a zone of inviolability – unlike the bodies of his subjects, which were vulnerable in all respects. Today every "real" body is perceived as "regal" – in itself removed from both material and symbolic violence. The fact remains, however, that this inviolability does not cover the entire human race but only one of its parts, to the detriment of the other. This is the other side of the immune paradigm, which is generally kept in the shadows. In terms of health and necessities, at least half of humankind is effectively deprived of the rights that, in theory, it should enjoy. This division is so obvious to everyone that there is no need to elaborate on it. Just consider the two opposing senses that the intensely immunitarian word "untouchable" assumes in different contexts: on the one hand, it designates someone protected from all possible threats; on the other, someone whom a society divided into castes pushes to its external borders, reducing the untouchable to a kind of human waste.

The immunization process splits into two opposing worlds divided by an impenetrable barrier, of which "apartheid" is simply the most extreme form, never entirely abolished. To grasp the nature of this phenomenon, whose proportions continue to grow, we must not lose sight of the thread that ties into a single knot the two human types involved. The two worlds – that of the untouchables and that of the inviolable – are not external to each other but complementary. It is not the case that some are protected while others are simply not. They are not protected in order to allow the others to be so. The preventive immunization of one group leads to the vulnerability of the other. The two conditions create an inversely proportional relationship: the more one group is immunized, the more the other is exposed to violence, discrimination, and abandonment. For immunity to be perceived qua immunity, it must, like any acquired right, always presuppose a segment of population that does not enjoy it – on social, economic, racial, or gender grounds. However far the dividing line shifts forward, inclusion can never become total; on the contrary, it tends to contract, to the benefit of exclusion. Each social function is cut and divided into two opposing parts, one internal and the other external. Just think of intercontinental travel, for example, which is divided vertically between the cruises of wealthy people in frantic pursuit of entertainment and the migration of poor people in desperate search of asylum. In this manner, instead of reuniting the divisions of caste, social rank, and class that separated premodern societies, modernity appears to inscribe them over and over within itself, separating different populations, but also different social strata within each population. For this reason, neither the rights declared to be "human" nor the legal category of "personhood" have succeeded in halting the dividing process; on the contrary, they have ultimately reinforced it through new exclusions. These *dispositifs* are legal and biopolitical at the same time; they operate on the border between inside and outside, opposing the protected and the exposed in constantly different ways.

From this point of view, although immunization reached full maturity during the modern age, it replicates the phobia of being touched, which Elias Canetti locates at the origin of human civilization; but it does so in an increasingly accentuated form.[4] Today more than ever, in the middle of a pandemic, when we measure even the distance between people in order to protect them from infecting each other, one senses a troubling relationship between origins and the present time that is paradigmatic rather than historical – with the difference that the masses, placed by Canetti at the pole opposite to individual distancing, are no longer an effective antidote. In fact our contemporary world is dominated by masses of individuals who are separated by *dispositifs* of communication and immunization at the same time. There is nothing more effectively disruptive of social relations than interconnection at any cost, to which we all seem to be devoted: it magnifies the isolation – or desolation – that appears to be the most widespread form of life today. Even technological tools such as videoconferencing are powerful creators of isolation, in the sense that they unite at a distance, thereby disuniting the people they ostensibly bring together. As we will see in relation to Niklas Luhmann, immunization is today's form of communication, exactly the way the language of communication is immunitarian. Instead of counteracting the civilizing process, this dynamic is its perverse effect. Similarly, in the semantic confusion that typifies our time, what we call "social distancing" is simply the other face of a global process in mass society that homogenizes lifestyles – partly because profound disparities lie beneath the surface homogeneity, but also because it expels those who lack the force to integrate.

It comes as no surprise that this process of desocialization, which affects all western democracies, has received an extraordinary boost in the time of the pandemic. During this period, what we define as biopolitics has taken on the outlines of a true immuno-politics. The prohibition against touching one another, which Norbert Elias identifies as one of the elements of the civilizing process, has become our form of life, along with the masks that hide the faces of people prevented from shaking hands when they meet. Meanwhile, video surveillance cameras monitor our movements and thermal scanners measure our body temperature. Italy is divided into zones of greater or lesser infection, indicated on a topographic map by colors of increasing intensity that block movements between impassable borders and obstruct physical encounters; and these are by now almost entirely supplanted by screen-based meetings. Even schooling – once an occasion for socializing, in addition to teaching and learning – takes place at a distance, or remotely, to use a term deliberately opposed to "proximate." Experience in common – of the *communitas* – thus becomes literally screened, divided by screens that prevent contacts, which are increasingly likened to contagions. In some countries there was even talk of shutting a segment of the "at-risk" population, primarily the elderly, in their homes and forbidding them to go out. The fact that the idea was not implemented does not mean that it will not be sometime in the future, definitively linking immunitarian democracy to the exclusionary *dispositif*.[5] Granted, these measures appear to have been superseded today by increasingly widespread vaccination and the arrival of new treatments after the onset of the disease. But there is no guarantee that the terrifying snapshot taken just a few months ago will not return sooner or later to imprint itself on our lives.

2

There is more to say, however, about the intrinsic connection between democracy and immunity, about democracy's immunitarian trait. As we have just seen, it can be described historically, starting with the first modern democracies and leading up to the hyperimmunitarian turn taken by democratic governments during the pandemic. But it can also be understood as a paradigm, tracing its roots to the very concept of democracy. This is what Jacques Derrida does in *Rogues*, written just after the September 11 attack on the United States. This was not the first book Derrida wrote about democracy. He had already approached the topic in different ways in previous works, from "Force of Law" to *The Politics of Friendship* and *The Other Heading*. The dominant idea in these texts was a deconstruction of the concept of democracy that tended to converge with the messianic notion of a "democracy to come." The latter bears traces of different meanings, ranging from the self-critical vocation of the democratic system to its limitless task, which is never reducible to a completed form. But something in *Rogues* appears to disable this promise, barring it from any possible historical realization: the awareness that a democracy in keeping with its name has never existed and will never be able to exist. For this reason, concludes Derrida, one cannot speak of democracy – at least not in the language that for two and a half millennia has tried to name it. Strictly speaking, democracy has no name; or rather no given content corresponds to the name "democracy": "Democracy is defined, as is the very ideal of democracy, by this lack of the proper and the selfsame."[6]

This void of meaning derives from the copresence in its lexicon of an irreconcilable dyad between the two poles of freedom and equality, but also within each pole. As for the first – freedom – ancient Greek philosophy identifies the prodromes of tyranny precisely in its ineluctable slide into license. Equality is also made problematic by the undecidable alternative between equal by number or equal by merit. This twofold tension produces a disintegrative force that contradicts the appeal to a democracy to come and takes the form of an inevitable self-destructive or self-immunitarian tendency: "What makes the aporia so formidable, and, it must be said, without any calculable, decidable, or foreseeable way out, [and] given over once more to the paradoxes of the autoimmune, is that equality is not equal to itself."[7] When the appeal to equality is reduced to a numerical calculation, as it is in democracy, the remedy proves to be worse than the disease: when it neutralizes natural disparity it ends up creating a new, more serious form of inequality. Oriented toward proportion, the appeal to equality leads to disproportion – this non-historical and therefore irremediable aporia is constitutive of democratic practice. By erasing the singularity of differences, democratic practice negates the equality of differences, thereby also negating democratic practice itself.

From here, then, comes the structurally autoimmunitarian character of *every* democracy. On the one hand, democracy opens a door to the incalculable and the immeasurable. On the other, it shuts it again, through a measurement that claims to be valid for all cases, regardless of the different starting conditions: "This chance is always given as an autoimmune threat. For calculating technique obviously destroys or neutralizes the incommensurable singularity to which it gives effective access."[8] Democracy is torn apart by two different, but also irreconcilable wills that are clearly in conflict: to welcome the excluded of all kinds within its borders (but this would mean that it no longer has borders; it would be borderless) and at the same time to include only those it declares to be "citizens," "brothers," or "persons," excluding all those who, on the basis of its own norms, are not. For good reason, modern democracy is indistinguishable from the nation-state, without which it is inconceivable. The possibility of a universal democracy, extended to all humanity, has never been seriously entertained in our philosophical tradition – not even by Kant, who in his cosmopolitical texts writes about a "universal republic" but not about "universal democracy."[9] The very idea of popular sovereignty is a meaningless expression for him, given that only a state can be, or have, a sovereign. True, Kant was not a democrat. But even the first and greatest thinkers of democracy, Rousseau and Tocqueville, despite their different intents, are united in declaring democracy unattainable, on the basis of its own premises. Democracy is necessary, yet impossible. For Rousseau, it is inapplicable to any human society; for Tocqueville, it is destined to degenerate sooner or later into its despotic opposite.

Derrida's main point, on which he insists, is not about democracy's imperfectability, though, but about its mortal struggle against itself, or more precisely about what he calls its suicide: "Democracy has always been suicidal."[10] The example he uses is Algeria, both colonial and liberated. Colonization and decolonization were, both, autoimmunitarian experiences. In the first case, French democracy entered into blatant contradiction with its own ideals, to the point of creating a civil war. In the case of the liberated Algeria, democracy was suspended at its most solemn moment, in the act of the electoral liturgy, blocked between the first and the second round by the not unjustified fear that the winning party, once in power, would abolish democratic rules and install a theocratic regime:

> To immunize itself, to protect itself against the aggressor (whether from within or without), democracy thus secreted its enemies on both sides of the front so that its only apparent options remained murder and suicide; but the murder was already turning into suicide, and the suicide, as always, let itself be translated into murder.[11]

This is not about the transition from democracy to tyranny, which the ancient Greeks interpreted in cyclical terms; nor is it about the historically irrefutable fact that fascism and Nazism both came to power through democratic procedures. Rather the autoimmune *dispositif* nests in the very heart of democracy. The suspension of free elections in Algeria means that it may be impossible to distinguish between democratic alternation and alternatives to democracy. What looms large is the irreconcilability between freedom and equality in a democratic system of government: to preserve equality, you must give up freedom; to implement freedom, you must give up equality. But, more fundamentally, the question that cannot be answered "democratically" is whether those who might undermine democracy should also be treated equally. It is true that the decision taken by democratic Algeria was not a definitive abolition of democracy but only its postponement, until the risks created by the fundamentalist parties had been averted. Setting aside the fact that postponing an evil is a typical immune process, what converts immunization into an autoimmunitarian practice is the evidence that, at least in some cases, democracy can protect itself only by negating itself. It could be objected, of course, that we are talking about an extreme situation. Still, how many times have states of exception – or emergency, at least – been declared in democracies, suspending democratic rules for reasons of *force majeure*, and not always for brief periods? This leads to the assertion that democracy is impossible, not only effectively but also ideally: "there is no absolute paradigm, whether constitutive or constitutional, no absolutely intelligible idea, no *eidos*, no *idea* of democracy.

And so, in the final analysis, no democratic ideal. For even if there were one, this 'there is' would remain aporetic, under a double or autoimmune constraint."[12]

This contradiction applies to what we defined as "democracy" a little over two centuries ago; but it also applies to the political system that received this name roughly 2,500 years ago. Not even an appeal to classical Greece, to which we still resort to reassure ourselves with a sort of extreme symbolic gesture, manages to loosen the antinomian knot wrapped tightly around a word that is equally aporetic and indispensable to us, because "democracy is, already in Greek, a concept that is inadequate to itself, a word hollowed out at its center by a vertiginous semantic abyss that compromises all translations and opens onto all kinds of autoimmune ambivalences and antinomies."[13]

3

There is no doubt that the system of government born in Athens with the name *dēmokratia* (originally *isonomia*) after Clisthenes' reforms was something out of the ordinary. For the first time in the history of the world, an attempt was made to erect a political dam against the asymmetry of power, making power visible and, at least in theory, accessible to all.[14] Furthermore, the absence of representative mechanisms created the conditions for a governmental experiment that later, after a series of misunderstandings, was described as "direct democracy": a correspondence, at least potentially, between the governing and the governed. But there are a number of problems, if not flagrant flaws, with this oft repeated and beloved story. To begin with, it must be said that in ancient Greek philosophy, literature, and historiography the democratic model so admired by the moderns did not enjoy that much credit. Apart from Herodotus, who has the Persian scholar Otanes pronounce a eulogy of democracy in opposition to his two monarchic and aristocratic interlocutors, and apart from Pericles' controversial Funeral Oration for the

Athenians fallen in the Peloponnesian War, reported by Thucydides, the opinion that generally prevailed in Greek culture was critical of democracy – starting with Plato and Aristotle, who associated it with political instability and the risk of drifting into tyranny.

Even apart from this view, it must also be said that in Periclean Athens the proclaimed democratic equality was confined to a rather slim number of citizens: free-born and not in slavery, male, adult, and economically self-sufficient – unlike the others, who were excluded not only from holding office but also from the voter list. The number of citizens thus amounted to a few tens of thousands in a population four or five times larger. But if we consider the two words whose combination gave rise to the name of democracy – *dēmos* and *kratos* – the concept's problematic issues prove to be even more pronounced. The meanings of *kratos* range from legitimate power to violent domination, while those contained in *dēmos* are no less heterogeneous and layered. The word refers on the one hand to the entire active population and, on the other, to its strictly popular part – to the majority made up of the poor, as opposed to the minority composed of the rich. This overlap between two non-coinciding meanings, later transferred into the modern concept of "the people," can be linked to the fact that in the Athenian assembly the vote of the numerically larger group counted for the totality of voters, giving rise to a striking statement in Herodotus (3.80.6): "for everything is in the power of the crowd" (*en gar tōi pollōi eni ta panta*, ἐν γὰρ τῷ πολλῷ ἔνι τὰ πάντα). Logically, the inclusion of everything under the most (the crowd) can correspond only to a complementary exclusion of "the few," evidently reduced to "the nothing."[15] This *reductio ad unum* that assigns all the power to one group, even if it is a majority, contains an element of violence that will never cease to plague the democratic principle, tilting it toward what will be called, much later, "the tyranny of the majority" – almost a predominance of *kratos* over *dēmos*, or, better still, a reciprocal incorporation of the two words that makes one the subject of the other. Of course, this *kratos* is never separate from *nomos*, which binds the exercise of its power to a set of shared rules; but these rules are such that they combine unity and exclusion in a manner that we will find radicalized in twentieth-century political philosophy. In a genealogy of democratic ideology, although not explicitly, Luciano Canfora links democracy and dictatorship – and not only philologically. Starting from the Preamble to the European Constitution's incongruous academic reference to Pericles' Funeral Oration, Canfora rescues this ancient text to its correct interpretation against ideological distortions. Thucydides' Pericles does not link democracy and freedom, as democratic rhetoric would have it; in fact he sets them in opposition, to highlight the positive exception of the Athenian model. In Pericles' day, adversaries of the popular government criticized Athenian democracy as an essentially liberticide system. Pericles responds to them that Athens does not lack freedom. However, he does not challenge the generally anti-libertarian character of democracy – on the contrary, he implicitly confirms it; hence the original sense of his words, distorted by the drafters of the Preamble: "'The word we use to describe our political system is *democracy* because, in its administration, it relates not to the few but to the *majority*.' . . . Pericles goes on: 'However . . . freedom reigns in our public life' (ii 37)."[16] As evidence of this, Canfora reminds us that later, too, in the Greek language of the Roman period, the word *dēmokratia* (from which came, late in the Roman period, a very rare noun, *dēmokratōr* – someone who exercised a kind of personal rule not unlike dictatorship) means dominion *over* the people more than dominion *of* the people. For good reason, in *Civil Wars* (II, 122, 514), Appian argues that Caesar and Pompey contended for *dēmokratia* – that is, for power in Rome. And later it appears that Dio Cassius defined the dictator Sulla using the same expression. Canfora can thus conclude: "At this point, *dēmokratia* and 'dictatorship' coincide."[17]

Four centuries before the principate of Augustus, Thucydides himself considered Pericles a *princeps* ("first, most distinguished one"), but one defined as *prōtos anēr*, "first man" – the meaning of which is at least close, if not identical, to that of tyrant. All this tends to recede from view today, or to have blurred outlines – in a framework that needs to find a noble prototype of modern democracy, without realizing that by doing so it draws even more attention to democracy's problematic character. From the outset, Athenian timocracy – a more accurate name for what we call "democracy" – shows a markedly immunitarian aspect: it is exclusionary on the basis of criteria of gender and demography, but also of racial lineage. To enter the restricted club of the equals, you had to be a free adult male, but you also had to be native-born, with an Athenian mother and father, which is to say pure-blooded. Furthermore, you also had to be militarily engaged in the defense of the fatherland, in a virtual identification between citizen and warrior – and this in turn implied the economic possibility of possessing armor and adequate means of self-support. Certainly the birth of the Athenian fleet created the need to find sailors and widened the circle of citizenship, but its core remained the army. The same applies to Sparta, which was less distant from its rival city than may seem; hence the enduring myth of Sparta in Jacobin patriot ideology. In Sparta as in Athens, despite its different political system, the decision-making heart of the city was the fighting corps. This explains the powerfully immunitarian root in what would come to be seen as the first democracy:

> In Athens free men reduced those who were not free to the status of non-persons, and after Solon ... an abyss opened up between freedom and slavery. This abyss was never bridged. As indicated above, in Athens the ratio of free men to slaves was one to four, or at least so it seems at certain times in the fifth and fourth centuries. The great mass of non-persons was indispensable to the functioning of the system, which for as long as it could lived off wars of plunder and imperial domination.[18]

Athens was undoubtedly a democracy, except that democracy should not be understood as generalized equality or freedom extended to all, but rather as a system of quite rigid social stratifications. The fact is that, at the end of the fifth century, a citizenship of about 30,000 adult males of military age, free and pure-blooded, rarely sent more than 5,000 men to the assembly. Elsewhere Canfora recalls a significant passage in Gramsci, from Notebook 13, titled "Number and Quality in Representative Systems of Government." Distinguishing between oligarchic and elitist critiques of parliamentary democracy, Gramsci challenges the idea that the law of numbers is the supreme standard of democracy and that therefore one vote is as good as another. Since a numerical count is solely the outcome of a process dominated at all phases by the hegemony of the elites,

> it is not true, in any sense, that numbers decide everything, or that the opinions of all electors are of "exactly" equal weight. Numbers, in this case too, are simply an instrumental value, giving a measure and a relation and nothing more. And what then is measured? What is measured is precisely the effectiveness, and the expansive and persuasive capacity, of the opinions of a few individuals, the active minorities, the élites, the avant-gardes, etc. – i.e. their rationality, historicity or concrete functionality.[19]

What elitist theoreticians from Mosca to Pareto – with whom Gramsci agrees in this case – grasp is that "only in appearance do numbers triumph in democracy."[20] Behind the rhetoric of equal opportunity, the self-representation of democracy conceals the domination of power groups that determine its direction. The issue in this case is not the tyranny of the majority: it is the tyranny of the minority. As Mosca had argued earlier in *The Ruling Class*, no member of the majority can resist the force of the elite minorities. Gramsci's conclusion was that "therefore, democracy, where intended as effective government of the majority, is something intrinsically illogical and unrealizable."[21]

4

Because of an irrepressible autoimmunitarian tendency, democracy cannot assert itself without negating itself, because it responds to two divergent needs, each of which, if pushed beyond a certain limit, may entail the suppression of the other and, along with it, the destruction of the democratic government itself. Historically, the dichotomy between popular sovereignty and representation predominates. Popular sovereignty means that the people are at the same time the subject and the object of the law that they themselves make. Representation means that, for the will of the people to manifest itself, it must pass through a process of being delegated to representatives nominated by the people but not bound by their mandate until they are in office. This is not a simple diversification of functions, but rather two fundamentally different models that cannot be reconciled, except at the cost of an act of coercion that calls into question the very nature of democratic government.[22] The contradiction, which traverses and destabilizes it, lies in the fact that the citizens declare themselves to be the actors of actions that are carried out by others in their place. This discrepancy makes it impossible for the two poles of the democratic lexicon to combine in an organic synthesis. The principles on which they are based – presence and absence, immediacy and mediation, identity and difference – are radically opposed. To make sense, the criterion of representation requires the representatives to be absent, while the criterion of identity presupposes the presence of the people at the time of deliberation. Thus, while representation leads to a division between those who govern and those who are governed, popular sovereignty presupposes their unification.

Through institutional models of greater or lesser sophistication, modern democracies have always sought a balance between these two opposing demands; in spite of this, the goal has never been reached, either in practice or theory. There is little awareness of this discrepancy among political analysts. On each occasion, a structural contradiction is attributed to contingent dysfunctions or to a misapplication of the rules that can be resolved by reforming the electoral system. What escapes notice is the problematic character of election itself as the keystone of democratic dialectics. Bernard Manin has reconstructed its genealogy, tracing it to an unresolved tension between democracy and representation.[23] Granted, they are not necessarily incompatible: in two and half centuries no democratic system has given up representative delegation, but at the cost of incorporating an aristocratic element that, in the long run, has undermined its internal coherence. The origin of this contradiction, which actualizes democracy only by turning it into an aristocracy, lies in choosing election over selection by lot in the assignment of public functions. And yet this choice is anything but obligatory. Contrary to what one might believe, throughout history the two mechanisms were not mutually exclusive, in fact they coexisted until one of them – selection by lot – left the stage for good, opening the way to the triumph of the electoral principle. In reality, selection by lot existed and sometimes predominated not just in Athens, the most ancient of democracies, but also in republican Rome and in Renaissance democracies, especially in Florence and Venice. It received serious consideration or was even preferred by authors such as Machiavelli, Guicciardini, Harrington, and Montesquieu, not to mention Rousseau. All of them established a close connection between selection by lot and democracy and grasped the essentially aristocratic character of election. In a passage from *The Social Contract*, as he cites Montesquieu, Rousseau states explicitly that selection by lot is "in the nature of democracy"[24] and, by contrast, places election on the side of aristocracy.

Just a generation later, what until then had been virtually a given – selection by lot, with its democratic nature – vanished from the horizon of possible options and appeared to be little more than an extravagance inherited from outdated political systems. Manin locates the source of this marked discontinuity in a conceptual transformation that, starting with the natural law jurists, views consensus as the only font of political legitimacy. Since selection by lot is impossible to relate to consensus, it ends up being obscured in favor of election, the most exemplary expression of consensus. This gives rise to a kind of historical conceptual paradox: just when the equality of citizens became a general principle, the mechanism most able to ensure it vanished in favor of an electoral *dispositif* destined to separate the electors from the elected. The debate, which foreshadows the United States Constitution (although with noticeable differences between federalists and anti-federalists), signaled the victory of election; and afterwards this result has never been challenged as a basic democratic process. France followed a similar, albeit revolutionary path. Against Rousseau's firm endorsement of direct democracy, Sièyes, like James Madison, sided with the representative model.[25] In *Considerations on the Government of Poland*, Rousseau declares representative delegation legitimate under certain geopolitical circumstances, but only if the representatives are strictly bound to follow the wishes of their electors and have the possibility of dismissing the appointed representatives if those stray from their instructions.[26] However, the difficulty of implementing this arrangement then tips the balance of the electoral process toward the aristocratic regime. Since there is no effective method for the electors to force the elected to follow their will, the only way to sanction them is by not voting for them in the next election. Only after having betrayed their mandate will they pay the price, through an early end to their political career. But this only accentuates democracy's squint: "it is by considering the past that voters are best able to influence the future."[27]

What lies behind this autoimmunitarian paradox of democracy – a system of government that can realize itself only if it becomes aristocratic by crippling its egalitarian principle? And what exactly are the aristocratic features of representative democracy? Since the beginning of the twentieth century, two factors above all have kept democracy's oligarchic destiny hidden from observers: the disappearance of census requirements for being elected; and the broadening of the electorate until universal suffrage was attained. But neither of these victories, which bear a clear democratic hallmark, has been sufficient to prevent democracy's drift toward aristocracy. Four basic reasons explain this outcome: the unequal treatment of candidates; the inevitable discrimination implicit in every choice; the advantage provided by certain characteristics of the candidates; and the cost of electoral propaganda, which only the more affluent can afford. Consequently, although the voters are equal, the same thing cannot be said of the candidates, who are increasingly remote from them. Those who get elected are not the ones most similar to the electoral body as a whole, but the least similar ones: "Since election involves a choice, it also includes an internal mechanism that hinders the selection of citizens who resemble others. At the head of the elective procedure, there is a force pulling in the opposite direction from the desire for similarity between rulers and ruled."[28]

This does not mean, warns Manin, that the electoral method lacks democratic elements – not only because every citizen's vote is as good as any other's, but also because voters can remove those who govern at the end of their term. It is just that the only people who can get elected are always those who have the greatest resources – and no one else. This means that, like Janus, elections have two faces: they are egalitarian and inegalitarian, democratic and aristocratic at the same time. This ambivalence pushes democracy outside its own boundaries, but it also forces it to assume characteristics typical of the aristocratic regime that, on paper, it opposes.

The only thinker to note this double-faced nature of elections, whether democratic or antidemocratic, was Carl Schmitt. In his *Constitutional Theory* he states explicitly: "In comparison to the selection by lot, that by election, as Plato and Aristotle correctly say, is an aristocratic method.

But it can appear as something democratic in comparison with the appointment by a higher organ or, indeed, to a selection by way of hereditary succession."[29] Whether one principle or the other prevails depends on the inclination of the electoral method toward the democratic pole of identity or toward the aristocratic pole of representation. As we shall see more clearly further on, the discourse splits into an alternative with no intermediary: an alternative not between two types of democracy but between a democratic and a no longer democratic system. For Manin, the contradiction is not external but internal to democracy – and to the electoral method that characterizes it, which is democratic and aristocratic at the same time: one within the other. Here we find the heart of democracy's autoimmunitarian *dispositif*. Democracy immunizes itself against excessive identification by means of an element foreign to its own mode of being; however, like an autoimmune disease, this element threatens to destroy it. The more democratic it is, the more aristocratic it is, too. The principle of representation's increasingly pronounced primacy over the principle of identity risks transforming democracy into its oligarchic opposite.

5

But the opposite choice, which sacrifices representation to identity, triggers an autoimmunitarian outcome as well. Its most illustrious interpreter – considered, quite rightly, to be the founder of modern democracy – is of course Rousseau. His relentless critique of representation – motivated by the argument that the general will "cannot be represented at all: either it is itself, or it is other; there is no middle at all"[30] – issued from the need to eliminate all separation between the source of sovereignty and its exercise. A true democracy is one in which people exercise sovereignty directly, since they are simultaneously the subject and the object of their own power. This comes about through the alienation of each associate from the community to which he or she belongs. In this way, "since alienation is done without reserve, the union is as perfect as it can be."[31] Hence, the famous passage on incorporation: "We each share our person and all our power under the supreme direction of the general will and, as a body, we receive every member as an indivisible part of the whole."[32] Once any distance between one another is eliminated in a "common self," individuals are fully immanent in the totality of which they are a part and from which they are no longer separable. All the divisions that create chasms in the social body – between the legislative and the executive, the public and the private, power and knowledge – are burned to the ground, in order to create an absolute identity. With the passing of the exteriority of representation, which pre-supposes the absence of the represented, there remains the pure presence of a community in perfect coincidence with itself. Inside the community – as Rousseau argues in *Emile* – a kind of metaphysical transposition takes place, "so that he [any man] no longer regards himself as one, but as a part of the whole, and is only conscious of the common life."[33]

Nevertheless, at the peak of identity – understood by Rousseau as the distinguishing feature of an authentic democracy – the split resurfaces: between individuals and the totality, between single subjects and the collective body. Despite Rousseau's harsh criticism of Hobbesian individualism, he remains within Hobbes' framework, seeking the precondition of community in the realm of nature, where humans live so divided that the risk of clashes between them is very low. Indeed, the greatest conceptual difficulty that Rousseau never managed to resolve is that of seeking to derive a philosophy of community from a metaphysics of solitude. In the communitarian model he advocates for the community of Clarnes, for example, the ontological intensity of the transition from an individual "one" to a collective "One" is such that it remodels human nature itself: "He who dares to institute a people must feel up to the task of changing human nature, so to speak: of transforming each individual, who is by himself a perfect and solitary whole, into a part of a bigger whole, from which this individual should somehow receive life and being."[34] From this point of view, those who glimpse a totalitarian germ in Rousseauian democracy – however dissimilar it may be to twentieth-century totalitarianism – perceive an undeniable component of his paradigm. Once all differences are abolished, nothing remains but a metaphysics of presence that seeks to fully homogenize all individual existences.

On closer analysis, this project, too, is not immune from internal contradictions, showing that, when the democratic system is deprived of one of its polarities – freedom – for the sake of equality, it runs the risk of inverting into despotism. The more Rousseau pushes toward the *reductio ad unum*, the more an internal fracture, both ontological and political, re-emerges as an unintended effect. While his autobiographical writings give ample evidence of this in their expression of an absolutely singular existential mode, his political writings call attention to a set of unresolvable contradictions. As the philosophical tradition has always demonstrated, the One is politically unrepresentable, except in totalitarian form. In politics, and especially in democracy, there is only the "two" – or at least a functional tension between distinct, heterogeneous institutions: between sovereignty and government, the legislative and the executive, knowledge and power. As for the first polarity, Rousseau himself argues that, while popular sovereignty is indivisible and inalienable, the exercise of power can be delegated to other bodies, even if through provisional and revocable mandates. Regarding the relationship between the legislative and the executive, in his opinion it would be better if they coincided, but a total overlap seems difficult to achieve, except under ideal conditions that are unlikely to occur together: a state of moderate size, with citizens who are virtuous and possess essentially equal economic resources. How can a people remain permanently united in assembly? And again, if it is true that whoever makes the law knows better than anyone else how it should be executed, "this is exactly what renders that government insufficient in some respects, because things that ought to be distinguished are not, and the prince and the sovereign, being nothing but the same person, make as it were only a government without government."[35]

To overcome these difficulties, Rousseau adopts the mythical solution of the divine legislator, thereby restoring the very transcendence he sought to avoid. The result is a twofold divergence that ultimately undermines the cohesiveness of his perspective. While the political mediation of the government may interrupt the sovereign people's self-determination of the law, the legislator's exteriority outside the social body breaks the community's self-referential circle with itself. This leads to the loss of its required perfect identity, causing it to relapse into the separation between the knowledge of those who create the law and the power of those who enact it. The source of this discrepancy is always an unresolved integration between the many and the one, but also a gap between command and obedience that arises from this failed integration. We know that Rousseau's solution is to make the people simultaneously subject and object of their own command. But in the meantime, before being constituted, what is a people if not a dispersed multitude? How can it make itself the constituent of itself, when it is not yet constituted? And can it constitute itself without a constituent act that gives it a political form? Admittedly, these questions presuppose the Hobbesian representative model, which Rousseau opposes to the concept of general will. But the issue is hardly resolved by this; it is simply shifted into that of the general will. What is in the general will to ensure that the conflict between different interests will be resolved without erupting again, stronger than before? Certainly, the general will eliminates the problem of consensus, radically modifying the paradigm of election-based democracy. From this point of view, Rousseau sidesteps the aristocratic tendency associated with the liberal theory of representative democracy. The general will is based on the people's immediate identification with itself: there is no consensual sharing or dialectical exchange between differing opinions.

This radical move, which turns the many into a single body politic, explains the future French revolutionaries' fascination with Rousseau. What they appreciated was not so much the stability of institutions as the exceptional shock force of a people moved against its enemies by a single will. Hannah Arendt notes that, unlike in American constitutionalism, in Rousseau's work the notion of "enemy" plays a decisive role. The concept is based on political experience, which teaches that only the presence of a common enemy can create a cohesive internal front that is otherwise prone to split: "Only in the presence of the enemy can such a thing as *la nation une et indivisible*, the ideal of the French and of all other nationalism, come to pass."[36] Needless to say, this presupposes the primacy of foreign policy, which thus becomes the prototype of all politics, as Saint-Just was careful to point out. But Rousseau's most original move consists in using opposition to shift the unification *dispositif* into the realm of internal politics. He identifies the common enemy as the particular interest and will of each individual – as opposed to the general interest and general will. Once will and interest are superimposed, they can be conceptualized in a perennial battle between the particular and the general.

Rousseau's stroke of genius – or fatal error, depending on your point of view – was to sum up all the particular interests and make them into a single inimical block from which he could draw, by opposition, the nation's *union sacrée*: "the oneness of the nation is guaranteed insofar as each citizen carries within himself the common enemy as well as the general interest which the common enemy brings into existence; for the common enemy is the particular interest or the particular will of each man."[37] Just as the common enemy consists of the sum of particular interests, the general will is equivalent to the sum of the renunciations that each individual makes toward him- or herself when becoming a citizen. "To partake in the body politic of the nation, each national must rise and remain in constant rebellion against himself."[38] This translation into politics – into war, actually – of the clash between individual and collective interests is the principle that unites the French and the communist revolutions despite their many differences and distinguishes them from the American Revolution, to which Arendt's approval goes instead. Her criticism of Rousseau targets his transposition of the "two-in-one" of thought into the conflictual "two-in-one" of the soul, which turns against itself out of compassion for the lowest people in society. This is the unrelenting clash between selfishness and pity, with which Rousseau replaces the solitude of the mind engaged in dialog with itself. The premise on which this substitution is based is that "the heart begins to beat properly only when it has been broken or is being torn in conflict."[39] The auto-immune *dispositif* takes center stage once again. When its discordant poles fall out of balance, democratic theory is ready to be turned into a theory of revolution, thereby negating its own nature. From this perspective, too, when democratic practice immunizes itself against its aristocratic tendency, it ends up self-destructing.

6

The most extreme interpretation of democracy's auto-immunization process was developed by Carl Schmitt, between the 1930s and the 1940s. In his theory, the contradictory elements identified so far in both ancient and modern democracy fuse into a self-disintegrative mixture that, as often happens with the German jurist, brings them into sharp relief and exacerbates them at the same time. The premise from which his analysis takes its cue is a clean break between the two contrasting poles of the democratic principle – freedom and equality, representation and identity, plurality and unity. For Schmitt, a rigorous theory of democracy rests not on their equilibrium but on their divarication. Contrary to the general tendency in political science to articulate democracy and liberalism into a single liberal–democratic regime, Schmitt clearly distinguishes between their respective rationales and outcomes. He judges the liberal mix of individualism and universalism, devoid as it is of any legitimating grounds, to be contradictory and ineffective, whereas democracy strikes him as our destiny – a challenge we cannot avoid. The same contrast makes opposites of the founding principles of the two systems of government. Although freedom per se is not the bearer of political form, equality does bring homogeneity to the people – on the condition, of course, that equality is not construed as generic parity between human beings but as the concrete identity of a people capable of political existence. This is the only way a people can express its constituent power, turning an indistinct multitude into a politically significant unit.

But how does the constituent power of a people not yet constituted manifest itself? This problem is similar to the one raised by Rousseau's *volonté générale*. Like the French philosopher, Schmitt does not accept the election mechanism, particularly via secret ballot, which he considers a privatization, and therefore a neutralization of political action. Nor does he have much confidence in parliamentary debate, which he regards as unproductive and incapable of decision-making. In his view, the only effective democratic act is the ancient Roman practice of *acclamatio*: "In fact, the real activity, capacity, and function of the people, the center of all popular expression, the original democratic phenomenon, what even Rousseau indicated as being a real democracy, is acclamation, the cry of approval or rejection from the united masses."[40] Contrary to those who consider acclamation an institution of the past that can no longer be revived, Schmitt sees in it the source of direct democracy – in other words, the only form of authentic democracy. After all, no past or present state has been able to do without it. Even a monarch needs an acclaiming people to clear the way, to publicly legitimize royal power: "acclamation is an eternal phenomenon of all political communities. There is no state without a people, and no people without acclamations."[41] Clearly, popular acclamation requires the presence of an acclaimed person: a general for the army, a leader for the people. The people approve or reject the proposal, knowing that they share the same political community. Without this act of identification, there could be no real democracy, but simply an addition of the individual opinions expressed privately in the voting booth. This leads to the apparently aporetic conclusion that democracy and dictatorship are not only compatible but also inextricably linked, which is unimaginable under the liberal regime. As Rousseau had done via the myth of the great legislator, Schmitt evokes the figure of the educator: he alone is capable of making the people recognize its own will. But this means adapting the democratic principle to the possibility of dictatorship. Schmitt does not underestimate the disruptive consequence of this admission: if democracy needs a dictatorship to form the people, then the democratic system can realize itself only by negating itself. "The consequence of this educational theory is a dictatorship that suspends democracy in the name of a true democracy that is still to be created."[42]

Never before had the autoimmunitarian potential of the democratic principle been exposed as it is here. Democracy can be accomplished only through the figure of its opposite. One has the impression that the connecting thread between democratic theory and democratic practice is stretched to breaking point. Even if democracy and dictatorship have opposite political methods, from a theoretical angle they do not exclude each other. Once the principle of freedom has been expelled from the framework of democracy, dictatorship makes its appearance as a possible outcome, if not as its fated fulfillment. Even under a dictatorship, a state can continue to define itself as democratic. Despite its liberticidal practice, bolshevism never stopped proclaiming its democratic status. When it suspended formal democracy in the name of a "substantial democracy," its totalitarian practice continued to appeal to democratic principles. After all, revolutionary democracy, theorized in its time by the Jacobins, led a minority to act in place of a majority – in the name of the general interest. Just as there can be parliamentarism without democracy, so there can be democracy without parliamentarism. Here is where any contact between Montesquieu and Rousseau breaks down. The theory that Montesquieu developed around the separation of powers, particularly of the legislature from the executive branch, does not fit into the picture of identity proclaimed by Rousseau. And in fact in the mid-nineteenth century dictatorship did return to the scene, in opposition not to democracy but to parliamentary constitutionalism – which makes 1848 a year of democracy and dictatorship at the same time, both being opposed to bourgeois liberalism. This applies all the more to twentieth-century mass democracy, which in terms of principles is even more remote from the liberal universe.[43] Whereas liberalism implies pluralism and difference, mass democracy presupposes unity and homogeneity. The problem raised by Schmitt is far from being resolved. He, too, finds it difficult to admit that, for democracy to be rescued from liberal neutrality, it must be delivered to dictatorship.

Schmitt would never succeed in getting to the bottom of this paradox. Its root lies in the "negativity" assigned to the idea of the people. Like any political concept, it, too, in Schmitt's perspective, acquires meaning from its opposite. The people is irreducible to any other political subject and can only be defined by negation. It is made up of "everyone who is *not* honored and distinguished, everyone *not* privileged, everyone prominent *not* because of property, social position, or education."[44] The "negative" status of the people is further intensified with the advent of capitalism. The people, or the proletariat, is the part of the population excluded from the ownership and production of surplus value. The only way the people can go beyond this negativity and assert itself positively is by assuming a public dimension and producing publicity by its very presence. Schmitt has no reservations about accepting Rousseau's idea that a people that is present cannot be represented: to be represented, it must be absent. But an absent people cannot be defined as a people, hence the recourse to acclamation as the only way for the people to manifest its presence. Certainly, admits Schmitt, we can imagine a future in which all citizens express their opinion from their own homes – today we would say through the Internet. But in this case there would be no public opinion, and therefore no general will but simply a sum of particular options – what Rousseau interpreted as the public enemy. It would be the end of democracy, which would slide into liberal privatization. Nevertheless, the author concludes: "The danger is not great as long as there is a substantive democratic similarity among the people, and as long as the people have political consciousness that can distinguish between friend and enemy."[45]

This identification of the people with the capacity to distinguish between friend and enemy must be kept in mind, because it forms the aporetic core of a perspective that brings democracy's autoimmune logic to a climax. Once again, Schmitt follows Rousseau's reasoning, also reconstructed by Arendt, but radically reverses her conclusion. Where she rejects the principle of exclusion, blaming it for the failure of the French Revolution, Schmitt adopts it as a mandatory step in democratic practice. He starts by observing that an absolute identity of all with all is in reality impracticable, at least from a legal point of view, since it would blur the distinction not only between judge and defendant but also between one party and another in a dispute. However, the most important thing is to avoid liberal neutralization, assuming that the criterion of similarity – the assimilation of like to like – is not enough to keep it at bay. Dissimilarity is also needed, which opposes one person, or several, to another. The two should not be juxtaposed but rather arranged in an essential correspondence, in the sense that the criterion for heterogeneity is what makes homogeneity possible. Democracy can be what it is only if, just as the similar is to be treated in the same way, the dissimilar is to be treated differently. The equality of the homogeneous corresponds to the distancing, in other words the exclusion, of the heterogeneous.

In addition to being a logical necessity, this is a historical fact. There has never existed a democracy, ancient or modern, that did not exclude a part of the population from political rights – by turns barbarians, atheists, aristocrats, counter-revolutionaries. Neither the Athenian democracy nor the Roman Empire nor the British Empire ever imagined granting equal rights to all the residents in their territories; not to mention colonial policies, which allowed European democracies to include in their dominion populations that were located outside their borders. The idea that every person has the same rights is liberal, not democratic. If democratic rights were to be applied indiscriminately to everyone, equality would be deprived of its essential meaning, which is conferred solely by the inequality of those who do not belong. This distinction – or, better yet, opposition – between equals and unequals, citizens and foreigners, friends and enemies – is precisely what defines the specificity of democratic politics: whoever does not belong to the state, like any foreigner, must be excluded. Consequently, in the theorization of the greatest political analysis of the twentieth century, democracy's autoimmune suicide is complete, because democracy is defined not by the principle of inclusion but by that of exclusion.

7

How can democracy escape the self-disintegrating fate that undermines it from within? Certainly not by imagining that it can cast off its immune *dispositifs* for the sake of an unattainable *communitas*. Like any body politic and any human body, it needs an immune system that can keep it alive, preventing it from precipitating into its opposite – into aristocracy or into despotism. The immune system is formed by the balanced copresence of the two opposing principles it comprises: equality and freedom, sovereignty and representation, unity and plurality. We have seen that the absolutization of one to the detriment of the other can lead a democratic government to a destructive end. When the liberal principle of separation between rulers and the ruled prevails, via representative delegation, democracy slides toward aristocracy. When the organic principle of popular sovereignty takes hold, there looms the opposite danger, that of despotism. In each case, democracy seems unable to withstand the impact of its own principles. The *reductio ad unum* of its two poles breaks down the complex mechanism on which it rests. From this point of view the problem is not, as is sometimes suggested, democracy's incompleteness, its broken promises, but, on the contrary, the attempt to achieve completeness through a drastic simplification of its internal dialectics.[46] Only if equality and freedom, popular sovereignty and representation, unity and distinction remain balanced can democracy avoid turning into what negates it.[47] Since it cannot fully assert itself through a single principle, it must necessarily incorporate its antidote, without, however, allowing itself to be overwhelmed by it. It administers itself a sustainable dose of negation, so to speak, in order to avoid larger negativity. This is the only way to stop its immune system from tipping over, in autoimmune terms.

But this position is inadequate. Or, better yet, it must be strengthened through the introduction of a third principle, which disrupts the exclusivity of the first two. To understand how it works, we must go beyond the classic opposition between the "Hobbesian model" – the source of representation – and the "Rousseauian model" – the source of identity – by way of a third landmark, which can be attributed to Tocqueville. I am referring to the associative principle he places at the base of American democracy, alongside the concepts of equality and freedom, interpreting them along the lines of what would be called institution-alism today. The space he devotes, in both editions of *Democracy in America*, to the practices of self-government created by American decentralization in contrast to French centralism is well known. Tocqueville writes that, "[i]n democratic countries, the science of association is the mother science; the progress of all the others depends on the progress of that one."[48] This is because – contrary to what Hobbes and Rousseau thought, each from his own angle of view – intermediate bodies, such as parties and associations, do not divide the country but rather unite it. Stimulating citizens' direct participation in local govern-ment, they create the necessary bridge between society and politics. Both sovereignty and representation are invigor-ated by it, which blocks the autoimmunitarian tendency. Sovereignty tempers the absoluteness of the majority prin-ciple to the advantage of minority rights. Representation attenuates the distance between the rulers and the ruled by engaging with social demands from below. This is why, Tocqueville continues, "Americans of all ages, all con-ditions, all minds constantly unite"[49] in consociational forms that, if organized, become institutions, alongside the parties. Indeed, the interests that they represent precede those represented institutionally by the parties, compared to which the associations are second-degree institutions, so to speak, because they respond not to the prescription of written laws but to customs, habits, and traditions that turn out to be no less binding. Although they differ from economic corporations, they are not expressed by the sov-ereign power – which, on the contrary, is amended and not infrequently undermined by them.

In twentieth-century political philosophy, Tocqueville's insights were developed primarily by Hannah Arendt. Like him, she too develops a twofold critique of the sovereign *dispositif* and of the mechanism of representa-tion. Regarding the first, she goes so far as to state: "In this respect, the great and, in the long run, perhaps the greatest American innovation in politics as such was the consistent abolition of sovereignty within the body politic of the republic."[50] Next, regarding representation, she cites Thomas Jefferson and argues that the goal of the American constituents was to encourage citizen participation in the government of public affairs not just once a year, during elections, but every day. She concludes that this goal was not reached – since in America, too, the representative government became an oligarchic government poised between democracy and aristocracy – but things were moving in the right direction. The direction consisted in placing, between sovereignty and individuals – which were locked in a two-way relationship under the *ancien régime* as well as under the revolutionary republic – a set of intermediate bodies whose purpose was to establish a plural regime: "These new body politics really were 'political societies,' and their great importance for the future lay in the formation of a political realm that enjoyed power and was entitled to claim rights without possessing or claiming sovereignty."[51] This arrangement already existed when the American colonies were subject to British rule. Once liberated, instead of losing autonomy, they implemented it in what was to become the federal government of the Union. By being maintained, these new political bodies were able to keep alive the dialectic between constituent and constituted power that was blocked in the transition of the French Revolution.

From here – since the drafting of the constitutions in the thirteen former colonies just before the Declaration of Independence – came a new conception of authority, embodied by representatives who, for their part, had been delegated from below. The extraordinary originality of the federal structure stemmed from the fact that its institution preceded not only the revolution but also colonization, given that it dates to the Mayflower Compact drawn up on the *Mayflower* and signed by the colonists when they landed in America. This meant that, in contrast to what happened in France, the revolution did not cast the rebels into a sort of state of nature; it allowed them to come together in a series of agreements and promises that remained intact after the liberation. As the ancient restorative meaning of 'revolution' attests, there is a mirror-image relationship between a new revolutionary regime and the one it overturns. The more absolute the sovereigns, the more absolutist the revolutions that depose them; these revolutions inherit their prerogatives, which are transferred from the monarchy to the nation. Sieyès did no more than "put the sovereignty of the nation into the place that had been vacated by a sovereign king."[52] Against this furious unification of all into one – which brought Rousseau's *volonté générale* into life – the American constituents discovered the principle of the divisibility of power and of the constitutive role of the opposition, understanding that political conflict strengthens rather than weakens democracy: "the recognition of the opposition as an institution of government . . . is possible only under the assumption that the nation is not *une et indivisible*, and that a separation of powers, far from causing impotence, generates and stabilizes power."[53] Only if structured in differentiated, independent institutions can the democratic system of government escape its autoimmunitarian tendency, which drives it along the old rut of aristocracy or onto the road of a new despotism.

In a recent book on democracy after decline,[54] Étienne Balibar, too, returns to the need to rethink together the three moments of representation, participation, and conflict. The divergent agreement between freedom and equality in the notion of *egaliberté* is not sufficient to jump-start the democratic machine, unless it is accompanied by the apparently contradictory dialectic of insurrection and institution. To push back against today's powerful dynamics of de-democratization, we must invent a new democratic practice and institutionalize political conflict. If we think that neutralization is democracy's worst autoimmune disease, then we must abandon the outdated conservative view of institutions and recognize that they offer a hotbed of possible conflicts against new forms of inequality and exclusion. Conflict should be seen not only as a tool for attaining democratic goals but also as the prime institution of democracy. Along these lines, as Machiavelli taught us, civil conflict is an integral part of the civilizing path. Conflict, swinging perpetually between the extremes of civil war and a simple pluralism of opinions, is the only way to politicize democracy and save it from its always incipient autoimmune tendency.

3

In the Time of Biopolitics

1

It is striking that during the pandemic period, just when biopolitics occupied our entire contemporary horizon,[1] a string of critical stances were taken against it. Even to an inattentive eye, all of Foucault's insights appear to have been validated today, and even outdone by reality – from the disciplining of individuals to the control of populations, from the unfolding of pastoral power to the politicization of medicine. Granted, measures of confinement and distancing like those implemented almost everywhere in recent months have their roots in the ancient practice of quarantine. But in the past that practice was never extended across entire countries for such long periods, partly because there was no healthcare policy comparable to our current system – just as there was no world health organization. Even during the decades of welfare government – especially in European nations – although the protection granted to citizens extended to healthcare, it was more social than biological in character. Everywhere in the countries affected by the virus – all of them, with very few exceptions – protection focused obsessively on biomedical issues. In the meantime, the pandemic shifted power relations between political parties, often deeply transforming them. Even the cleavage between left and right, which for the past two centuries has been about social and civil issues, shifted conspicuously toward biopolitical matters – starting with the seeming alternative between health or freedom, both of which are guaranteed by modern constitutions.

But the biopolitical effects of the pandemic went well beyond competition between political parties, dragging in the relationship between politics and society and between institutions and protest movements, at times putting them at odds. At the same time, within governments, biopolitical effects altered the balance between the legislative and the executive to the benefit of the latter, sometimes with disruptive consequences. It is no mystery that the most important electoral contest in the world – for president of the United States of America – was heavily influenced by the presence of the virus; it probably overturned the expected results, before irrupting into the political arena. Domestic politics was not its only sphere of influence either. Its effects weighed on the European Union's political economy, which passed in a matter of months from a strenuous defense of the Maastricht criteria to the greatest enlargement of non-repayable funds ever recorded. It also altered relations between the great powers – first and foremost, the United States and China, which had already locked horns over the origins of the virus. But their confrontation shifted rapidly to vaccine production, in a relentless competition that soon enmeshed Russia, the United Kingdom, and Germany. It now seems quite likely that global geopolitical balances of power will be profoundly influenced by this competition, in a framework that affects countries but also relationships between public and private, funding and research, and knowledge and power. Given that the competition is not only about vaccine effectiveness but also about the space and time of their production and distribution, it can well be said that biopolitics has become the new transcendental horizon within which our entire contemporary experience revolves.

Despite this, or perhaps for this very reason, there has been a conspicuous distancing from the biopolitical paradigm in the cultural debate. Multiple rationales have been put forward, but the polemic proceeds mainly along three lines of argument: the lexical indeterminacy of the paradigm, its historical fragility, and its naturalist turn. As regards lexical indeterminacy, there is little doubt that the paradigm's growing success in different domains – from ethics to economics, technology, and ecology – may have slackened its conceptual contours. The different and sometimes opposing interpretations that the concept has received in philosophical discussion must also be taken into account, as they caused it to stray, quite far even, from Foucault's original configuration and weakened its theoretical status. Jean-Luc Nancy in particular was critical about its use from the beginning. He noted that, "as often happens, this neologism is also paying the price of success: nobody knows anymore what it means exactly."[2] François Warin, who inspired Nancy's polemic, was speaking of biopolitics thus: "this notion, is it not one of variable geometry, and hence not very consistent and with reduced functionality?"[3] Foucault originally confined biopolitics to the transformations of power during the eighteenth century, but bit by bit it was generalized, to the point of becoming "the war machine of alter-globalization fights"[4] fashioned by Michael Hardt and Toni Negri.

In reality, this highly idiosyncratic interpretation got its start from the antibiologist bias of Heidegger, for whom human life can be expressed only in terms of existence: against any immanentist hypothesis of simple survival, life must be exposed to something that goes beyond it. According to this critique, simple survival is exactly where Hobbes' biopolitical turn would lead – the turn he first introduced into the philosophical tradition when he made the preservation of life the epicenter of the political horizon. Since then, says Warin, the concept has been pulled off course in two directions: the first empties politics of its properly political content; and the second drags life down from the existential level of *bios* to the material level of *zoē*, losing the meaning of both in the process. Hence his assertion that "what theorists today call 'biopolitics' has nothing to do with either life as *bios* or politics in its Aristotelian and Greek definition; it would be more appropriate to call it zootechnics or ecotechnics."[5]

These are exactly the terms that Nancy uses to evacuate biopolitical semantics of its meaning: "Life as studied by biology can however concern zoology, physiology, neurology ... everything you want except what we define as 'the life of human beings,' that is, their existence."[6] As Heidegger argued back in the 1930s, politics, in its turn, has moved from the *polis* to the command-and-control centers of the ecotechnological complex, losing any distinctive qualities in the process. According to this narrative, biopolitics has merely completed the journey of depoliticizing politics and biologizing life that began in the nineteenth century. Nancy's conclusion, not unsurprisingly, is that "what we need lies today outside politics and certainly even outside life."[7]

This first line of criticism is flanked by another, equally fierce attack, which challenges biopolitics' untenable lack of historicity. For Paolo Flores d'Arcais, who represents the most vehement version of this offensive, biopolitics is "a paradigm that merely hints at its meaning; it is vague, manipulative, chaotic, and ungraspable, because it is at odds with all the historical data."[8] Owing to its conceptual approximation, Foucault's opposition between sovereignty and biopolitics would end up concealing the much more historically relevant contrast between the *ancien régime* and the modern democracy birthed by revolution. In this way the abstract concept of biopolitics, which can be made to encompass equally all systems of government and events of the past four centuries, would efface the distinction between reaction and revolution, absolutism and democracy, heteronomy and autonomy. Moreover, as Carlo Galli adds, with a sharper eye for historical–conceptual distinctions, Foucault takes his place in the tradition of negative thought, which, starting with Nietzsche, sees reality as a single forcefield in conflict that fuses all differences in a deconstructive vortex: "for indeterminate negation, everything can ultimately be equal to everything else, on a night when all the cows are black."[9] However, the dehistoricization process set in motion by biopolitical thinkers is said to produce an even more serious contradiction: it subjugates itself unconsciously to what it seeks to oppose. Once the logics of power have been extended to the totality of human relations, including the fields of knowledge that interpret them, there would be no opening left for criticism, which is doomed to slip into a kind of inert, acritical condition. This would explain the alignment with neoliberalism that some have sought to discern in Foucault's courses on biopolitics in the late 1970s: "The idea that power is within thought implies that thought is within power. Immanence has its own traps: Foucauldian criticism believes that it understands the *dispositifs* of power, and it is caught up in them to the point of not seeing, or of not seeing clearly, the contradictions that power does not want to show."[10]

These two critical perspectives are accompanied, finally, by a third one, which claims that the biopolitical discourse leads to a naturalistic and dehistoricized notion of life. In this view, the origin of this metaphysical deviation is, again, the missing connection between the regimes of sovereignty and biopolitics, which are set against each other without much reflection. Once sovereignty is placed under the banner of death and biopolitics is placed in an economy of life, Foucault's attention would concentrate on the latter, overlooking equally important topics related to modes of production, class struggle, and constituent and constituted powers. This would lead to a kind of "pan-biopoliticism" that flattens historical specificities into a single biological mold. By eliminating contradictions that run through society along lines irreducible to a single dimension, Foucault would turn events into simple predicates of a metahistorical universal devoid of any internal scansions. The accusation returns of reducing *bios* – the forms of life – to a *zoē* fixed to the eternal repetition of its natural status. Life, deprived of historical context, would remain imprisoned in a biological cage that cancels out the rhythm of existence. According to this critique, after drastically separating the two semantic blocks of life and death, Foucault – and biopolitical thought along with him – make it difficult to recognize the segment that connects them in perpetually changing forms, with the consequence that we lose sight of the ways in which different societies work in the concreteness of their processes. By claiming to be the only face of modern politics, biopolitics would cancel out all other perspectives, precluding itself from entering a critical relationship with our time.

2

In truth, if we read Foucault in an unbiased manner, none of these criticisms appears to be well founded; nor does the argumentative plot underlying them. As it turns out, the idea that his perspective lacks historicity, sliding into a kind of metaphysics of life, is contradicted by others – at times the same people – who criticize him for the opposite reason. For example, as Derrida argued, and in this he was followed by Nancy himself, Foucault is not a real philosopher but a cultural historian. This way of thinking takes for granted that there are no intrinsic relations between history and philosophy; on the contrary, there is a kind of contrast of principle between them. Now, if there is one thing that Foucault contests, it is precisely this assumption; it comes laden with heavy metaphysical collateral. Of course, once he places his own work at the intersection between philosophy and history, he makes scarce mention of the history of philosophy – for which he substitutes a genealogy of forms of knowledge

– and even less of any kind of philosophy of history. In reality, history has neither a predefined outcome nor a single origin in Foucault's view. If it had one or the other, there would be a point outside historicization, an ending or a beginning, posited as an absolute on which history itself is founded, going backward or forward. Rather he observes, "historical sense can evade metaphysics and become a privileged instrument of genealogy if it refuses the certainty of absolutes."[11]

Nothing escapes the grip of history – "we are doomed historically to history," writes Foucault in *The Birth of the Clinic*[12] – not only in the sense that every theory, like every practice, is inscribed within history, but also in the more conspicuous sense that each practice is created by history. The peculiar object of Foucault's study is not facts or concepts in themselves, but the condition of their historical emergence, the space–time context that leads to their particular configuration.[13] This occasions a radical change in what is commonly understood as "history" and "philosophy." It is as if philosophy, in the absence of an internal truth, had no content outside history; but this is a history shaped by a thought that formulates it according to the guiding truth of the time. With a single gesture, Foucault is able to escape from traditional historicism and from determinism: from historicism, because a later truth is not necessarily superior to an earlier one; and from determinism, because there is always a moment when the subject can remove itself from the process in which it is embedded, opening a new vector of meaning. This is not to say that we can exit history – where would we go? Rather it means that we can inhabit history differently, by adopting a critical attitude that is situated in the present but is able to contest it, by orienting it in a different direction. From this point of view, variation, which is always possible, does not involve the object of knowledge so much as the subject who formulates it. Even though we are always located in a historical constellation, we can modify it by creating friction with our conditions of existence.

Admittedly, Foucault employs this "existential" lexicon primarily in his later years, in parallel with his work on subjectification processes. But during his biopolitics period, too, contrary to the claims of his critics, Foucault's concept of "life" never coincides with the simple biological dimension. Even when taken in its materiality, life is never just itself – it is always filtered conceptually by the knowledge that questions it, removing it from absolute immanence. As early as 1971, during a debate with Noam Chomsky on the concept of human nature, Foucault stated that "the notion of life is not a *scientific concept*; it has been an *epistemological indicator* of which the classifying, delimiting and other functions had an effect on scientific discussions, and not on what they were talking about."[14] Contrary to those who accuse him of naturalizing life, he historicizes the idea of nature itself, tracing its beginnings to a certain phase in our civilization that was marked by particular cultural, political, and social conditions. By so doing, Foucault does not mean to deny that human nature is bound by a set of constants that place insurmountable limits on it. But he locates these limits outside rather than inside the human mind, "somewhere else, even outside the human mind," as Chomsky does, and precisely "in social forms, in the relations of production, in the class struggles, etc."[15] Part of the reason why he does so is that the body is not subject solely to the laws of physiology: it is shaped in all its extension by the historical regimes to which it belongs. Far from confirming the accusation that he biologizes human life, Foucault believes that the body is caught up in history, which penetrates inside it: "'effective' history deprives the self of the reassuring stability of life and nature."[16] True, at times life has undergone a biologizing process meant to crush it into its material layer; but that has happened precisely under the regimes – biopolitical or thanatopolitical – that Foucault criticizes, reconstructing their genealogical matrix. The biological naturalization he explains does not represent his perspective: it is the work of a biopower interested in controlling a life that becomes all the more inert the more it is biologicized.

Certainly the biopolitical paradigm bears this ambivalence inside: it is a process that Foucault captures in reality and, at the same time, the category that defines it conceptually. Thus, instead of reproducing a natural reduction, it introduces an artificial fold into nature. For Foucault, the concept of life has a precise historical matrix, but so do the forms of knowledge that brought it into being over time, starting with biology. Darwin did not intend to replace history with "metaphorizing history on the analogy of life,"[17] but intended to capture in life the signs, fractures, and resources of history; hence his idea that "life evolved, that the evolution of living species is determined, to a certain degree, by accidents which might be of a historical nature."[18] The biopolitical paradigm simply brings this principle to awareness, expressing the tension that simultaneously unites and opposes it to its object. For good reason, it has been associated from the beginning with "bio-history," with which it shares an inescapable interference between life and history:

> If one can apply the term *bio-history* to the pressures through which the movements of life and the processes of history interfere with one another, one would have to speak of bio-politics to designate what brought life and its mechanisms into the realm of explicit calculations and made knowledge–power an agent of transformation of human life.[19]

In this way, something taken as an unchangeable given – in Anglo-American theorizing on biopolitics, for example – became a problem situated at the crossroads of historical tangents, which are also able to be reconstructed historically. It is as if history – the point of view engendered by history – reverses the "natural" perspective imposed by biopower and rescues life from being flattened into nature, projecting it in different directions from one time to the next. If we consider the genetic variations of different populations, for example, "[h]istory designates these ensembles before erasing them; we must not look at them as raw and definitive biological facts that impose themselves, from the basis of 'nature', on history."[20] Obviously, life is not history – there is always a biological nucleus in it or a physiological margin that resists complete historicization and positions itself at its confines. But, from another point of view, this very exteriority is absorbed into the horizon of understanding opened by history. The most powerful meaning of biopolitics – misunderstood equally by its glorifiers and by its disparagers – is to be sought "in this dual position of life that placed it at the same time outside history, in its biological environment, and inside human historicity, penetrated by the latter's techniques of knowledge and power."[21]

The distinction between different regimes is subject to the same tension between correspondence and discrepancy, continuity and discontinuity. This starts with the distinction between sovereignty and biopolitics, crucial to Foucault, which has attracted the polemical attention of his critics. How are the two related? Do they follow each other or do they overlap? Are they heterogeneous or do they coexist? And how much of one remains inside the other, once it has been replaced? It must be said straightaway that Foucault does not answer these questions with clarity; it is as if he remained undecided between one hypothesis and the other – sometimes he switches, even in the same text, between two inconsistent interpretations. However, to fathom the issue in all its problematic depths, we must keep in mind two factors. The first is that, instead of approaching each era directly, he uses one to define the other by negation. Just as he did earlier in *Madness and Civilization*, defining the classical period through contrast with the Middle Ages, and in *The Order of Things*, positioning the modern episteme on the edge of the previous one, he carves out the contours of biopolitics from the negative mold of sovereignty, although without opposing them point by point. On the contrary, what draws Foucault's attention is precisely the moments in which sovereign power reemerges in the biopolitical field, almost like a ghost, and introduces the production of death into the expansion of life. This is where the second factor comes into play, driving Foucault's discourse in an apparently aporetic direction, namely toward the paradigmatic turn he impresses on his historical periodization. Both the concept of "sovereignty" and that of "biopolitics" should be understood not only as epochs but, in addition, as paradigmatic blocks not bound to a specific temporal threshold – namely, as perspectival axes that can project their lexicon beyond a given chronological horizon, linking the original to the actual, as it were. For example, just as the power to "give death" passed from absolute monarchies to a regime like the Nazi one, set in full biopolitical times, so too the paradigm of government that originated in the seventeenth century relocates – with adaptations, of course – to our liberal societies. When looked at from this perspective, then, no matter how staggered in time sovereignty and biopolitics are, they are also "contemporaneous," in the literal sense of the word: antinomically present at the same time.

3

In reality, the idea widely shared by Foucault's critics, that he abandons historicity to the point of making biopolitics a metaphysics of life, arises from a reading that is more incomplete than wrong. The first reception of Foucauldian biopolitics, swayed to some extent by the order in which his posthumous works were published, was based on the last chapter of *The Will to Knowledge* (volume 1 of *The History of Sexuality*) and on the last lecture of his 1976 Collège de France course, entitled "Society Must Be Defended." But this lecture was isolated from the others and, instead of being read as a conclusion to the project he had developed during the whole academic year, it was taken almost as a separate piece, as a source – in conjunction with the pages from *The History of Sexuality* – from which one could deduce Foucault's concept of biopolitics. What got lost in this process was the intrinsic relationship of the biopolitical paradigm with the historical perspective that the 1976 course opened; and the loss had strong dehistoricizing effects. From the very first lesson, in fact, Foucault argued that we must free the notion of power from its primarily juridical interpretation, in order to recognize its essentially historical nature, which is marked by an essential relationship to war. When thought of historically, politics turns out to be the expression of power relations as they are determined by current conflicts.

This polemological interpretation of politics – which replaces Wilhelm Reich's "power as repression" with Nietzsche's "power as war" – runs throughout Foucault's course, including the final pages on biopower. The premise on which these pages are based is the contrast with the sovereign *dispositif* that, as we know, characterizes Foucault's definition of biopolitics from the beginning. To analyze power away from the "Leviathan model" means to uncouple it from the tripartite model of subject, unity, and law, to which the concept of sovereignty destines it, and to bring it back to its irreducibly conflictual aspect. It is true that political power relations and relations of war should not be confused, but since relations of war express the utmost tension between rival parties, only they allow us to grasp the deeper nature of social dialectics. This is not because there is no state of peace – a destination to which all political systems lay claim – but because peace too, surreptitiously, speaks the language of war, from which in the final analysis it derives. In the same way, the legal order is merely the contingent equilibrium of a conflict destined sooner or later to re-erupt. State, law, and institutions are still the specific places of modern political action. But, instead of eliminating the inevitable discord that comes before and after them, all they do is momentarily neutralize it. For good reason, then, the most solid state institution, the one designed to influence the functioning of all the others, is the military. Today this original, never extinguished substrate of political relations is hidden from our view by the juridical conception of power elaborated in modern political philosophy, which is still dominated by the Hobbesian lexicon of state unity. This conception has ultimately effaced the irremediably binary nature of the social body – which was brought to light by the historical political discourse whose genealogy Foucault traces.

Still undeveloped in Machiavelli and negated by Hobbes, this discourse appears after the religious and civil wars of the sixteenth century. Formulated by the Puritans at the beginning of the English revolution, it re-emerged in France a century later, at the end of Louis XIV's reign, but with opposite intentions. Employed in England against the monarchy – by political groups that represented the bourgeoisie and the lower classes and were led respectively by Sir Edward Coke and John Lilburne – it acquired the function of an aristocratic rearguard in France, through authors such as Boulanvillers and Fréret, and was finally incorporated into the nationalist perspective of Sieyés, Thierry, and Fréret. The link between such different political positions – revolutionary and reactionary, leftist and rightist, monarchical and republican – resides in an opposition to the pyramid model of the medieval era and to Hobbes' monism, but also to the tripartite order of society based on the estates of the *ancien régime*. The war *dispositif* counters them with a binary image of the social body, etched into the life of peoples by the succession of conquests and invasions, dominions and subjugations, pacts and betrayals that punctuate western history, starting with the fall of the Roman Empire. Foucault insists that this is the first rigorously historical–political discourse, in which the speaker, although representing the law, always sides with one party against the other, without ever taking a position in the center – as does, by contrast, the sovereign discourse. In a sequence of events from long ago but continually revived, in which strengths and weaknesses and victories and defeats square off, history acquires an immeasurable depth, a depth that cannot be contained within the limits of institutional order and dynastic legitimacy:

> it is a discourse that develops completely within the historical dimension. It is deployed within a history that has no boundaries, no end, and no limits. . . . It is interested . . . not in referring the relativity of history to the absolute of the law, but in discovering, beneath the stability of the law or the truth, the indefiniteness of history. It is interested in the battle cries that can be heard beneath the formulas or right, in the dissymmetry of forces that lies beneath the equilibrium of justice.[22]

When discussing the emergence of royal relations behind the curtain of legal representation, Foucault explicitly sings the praises of historicism – of course not in the name of continuism but, on the contrary, in the name of the continual contradictions that pull apart the story power tells of itself: "We must try to be historicists, or in other words, try to analyze this perpetual and unavoidable relationship between the war that is recounted by history and the history that is traversed by the war it is recounting."[23]

But what is the connecting link between this historical–political discourse (the first in the West, Foucault insists) and biopolitics? It is the racism that, at a certain point, guides the ancient struggle between different ethnic groups toward an intensely biological semantics. Starting in the early modern age, whoever takes a position in a battle, no matter on which side, does so in defense of a race and in opposition to another race. This lexicon, at once historical and natural, political and biological, varies in form from one time to the next, depending on the phases and contexts through which it passes. Two centuries after its inception, in the early 1800s, it split into two intertwined but distinct strands. On the one hand, the race struggle turned into a class struggle that incorporated racial elements but channeled them in a revolutionary direction. On the other, through Darwinian evolutionism, the race struggle solidified biologically, first serving nationalism and later colonialism. Foucault identifies the outcome of this process as a "statalization of the biological," which occurred when the two opposing races merged into a single national race in each state. That race then split again into two subraces, one dominant and the other dominated, and the latter was accused of degenerating and endangering the former's life. From then on, although racism never lost its outward-facing aggression, it also became an inward-facing *dispositif* of segregation and exclusion. According to it – states Foucault, echoing the title of his course – defending oneself against society is no longer the issue; on the contrary, "[w]e have to defend society against all the biological threats posed by the other race, the subrace, the counterrace that we are, despite ourselves, bringing into existence."[24]

This dialectic is the vitalist outcome, but also the lethal point of explosion, that arises at the confluence of two vectors, one historical–political and the other medical–biological. At a certain point they intersect, giving rise to two distinct but complementary technologies: the disciplining of individuals and the regulation of populations. The same relationship between sovereignty and biopolitics, never fully clarified by Foucault, receives a more convincing explanation here. Rather than two opposing regimes or two successive *dispositifs*, they appear to be operators of a single biohistorical complex that arranges them in layers. The first sovereign period, lasting until the second half of the eighteenth century, was followed by another, which was predominantly biopolitical and oriented toward the defense and development of individual and collective life. When biological racism crept into it, though, what used to be two different models crossed paths – with devastating effects. Into the biopolitical dynamic of defending life there crept a new sovereign power of "giving death." Racism not only delineates, within life, the threshold beyond which it must die; it also establishes an inversely proportional relationship between the life of some and the death of others. The death of the inferior race makes the life of the superior race healthier and purer. Racism is the condition that makes a politics of death possible, grafting it onto the trunk of the old nationalism. Having reached its paroxysmal culmination in Nazism, it conferred on the state the power of life and death over others; but it also granted this right, potentially, to each individual. Everyone was entitled to give death to their neighbor by making a simple complaint. In the name of the chosen race, at the moment of defeat, Hitler enjoined the entire German people to die, completely blurring the distinction between homicide and suicide:

> There was, in Nazism, a coincidence between a generalized biopower and a dictatorship that was at once absolute and retransmitted throughout the entire social body by this fantastic extension of the right to kill and of exposure to death. We have an absolutely racist State, an absolutely murderous State, and an absolutely suicidal State.[25]

4

As already mentioned, the historical depth of Foucault's discourse does not go against his philosophical bent. His placement of war at the heart of modern society in *Society Must be Defended* resulted from a theoretical move that radically changed the usual perspective of historiography. And yet, at the beginning of the course that followed – *Security, Territory, Population* – Foucault felt compelled to emphasize that what he was doing "is not history, sociology, or economics. However, in one way or another, and for simple factual reasons, what I am doing is something that concerns philosophy."[26] In what sense? What does Foucault mean when he explains: "it's up to me . . . to know on what fields of real forces we need to get our bearings in order to make a tactically effective analysis. But this is, after all, the circle of struggle and truth, that is to say, precisely, of philosophical practice"?[27] Before proposing an answer to this question, we must address the still unresolved issue of the relationship between the two courses and the noticeable terminological differences between them. The problem, as it has been framed by critics thus far, concerns the apparently abrupt and insufficiently motivated transition from the analysis of power still used in the 1976 course to the semantics of government begun in the 1978 course. At stake is the definition of biopolitics, sketched out at the end of *Society Must Be Defended* and apparently abandoned in favor of the new paradigm of "governmentality." But did he really abandon biopolitics? Why, in that case, when introducing the new course, would he propose: "This year I would like to begin studying something that I have called, somewhat vaguely, bio-power"?[28] And why, if he considered the topic closed, did he name the next year's course *The Birth of Biopolitics*? Put simply, as Michel Senellart asks in the epilogue to the 1978 course,[29] does the philosopher set off in a new direction, or does he inscribe the concept of biopower in a broader, more articulated framework?

Although history, sociology, and economics do appear in these lectures, Foucault's insistent references to philosophy may provide us with a key for approaching the problem and for understanding which "force field," as he calls it, to place it in. In reality, when Foucault introduces a new lexicon of government, he is not erasing the power theme: he is displacing it, moving it to an external sphere in order to be able to frame it from a different angle. After all, if there is something that describes Foucault's thought in spite of, and within, his continual metamorphoses, it is precisely his penchant for the "outside," as he titled one of his most powerful essays.[30] Each paradigmatic transition in his work is marked by a shift toward an ever greater exteriority, which, far from dissolving the object of study, maintains a relationship with it and reveals a facet previously left in the shadows. It is as if, to investigate something, Foucault opens an outside space from which to return to the object from its reverse side, so to speak, with a visual acuity not permitted by a frontal perspective. This is what happens to madness in *Madness and*

Civilization, when it is looked at from outside the field of reason, and to humanity in *The Order of Things*, when it is removed from the order of representation and examined, on the verge of its incipient disappearance; let alone what happens to statements, which in Foucault's lecture "The Order of Discourse" have been "restored" "to their pure dispersion," so as to be "analyzed" "in an exteriority that may be paradoxical since it refers to no adverse form of interiority."[31] Regarding these, anyone who speaks "is necessarily caught up in the play of an exteriority."[32] Every form of knowledge, for that matter, is questioned in relation to its presumption of truth, from the point of view of the powers in which it is embedded and from which it is ultimately constituted.

But, to go back to our starting question, this also holds for power in its specifically political dimension: Foucault submits it to the same estrangement method, by opening an analytical field that is heterogeneous, though not extraneous to it. He actually talks about this with regard to disciplining: "When in previous years we talked about the disciplines, about the army, hospitals, schools, and prisons, basically we wanted to carry out a triple displacement, shifting, if you like, to the outside, and in three ways."[33] The first displacement is a decentering away from what Foucault defines as "the 'institutional-centric' approach."[34] For example, he shows that the only way to comprehend the hospital structure is by starting from something more general, such as the psychiatric order. One must bypass the institution itself to bring into relief, in the background or behind it, the technology of power that regulates its functioning. Foucault's second decentering consists in creating a passageway from the institution to the outside. Regarding the prison, for example, he observes that its history is not marked by reform projects but by strategies made necessary by its institutional shortcomings. The third and final distancing concerns the object of study itself – delinquency, sexuality, population – which is removed from its immediate visibility and brought back to its genesis. At this point, however, he finds himself faced with a new problem: to escape from individual institutions and backtrack to the technologies that produce them means re-entering by another route the more general space from which they receive their lifeblood, namely the state horizon.

The only way to prevent this short circuit is to look at the state from the outside, too, by opening a space external to it. This is not to negate its reality – which would be impossible – but to place it in a broader and more complex framework, without allowing oneself to be blinded by its solitary myth. This non-statal space, out of which the state issues, is governmentality. Far from replacing the notion of biopolitics in Foucault's conceptual lexicon (as has been argued), governmentality is a specific historical instance of biopolitics, so much so that he asks: "Can we talk of something like a 'governmentality' that would be to the state what techniques of segregation were to psychiatry, what techniques of discipline were to the penal system, and what biopolitics was to medical institutions?"[35] We do see a perceptible change in Foucault's argumentative strategy, since his aim now is to convert the paradigms he had identified previously into the actual practice of modernization processes. Likewise, the dominant role assigned to war disappears. But this reinforces rather than effaces his allusion to life as power's domain of impact. From this standpoint, it could be said that the relationship in history between governmentality and the state is mirrored in the paradigmatic correspondence between biopolitics and sovereignty: governmentality is the exteriority that goes beyond the confines of the state while at the same time encompassing it. It is as if Foucault traced two genealogical lines, separate and joined at the same time, which overlap at a certain point, producing an altering effect from which modern politics has yet to free itself. The only ground on which modern politics can express itself does not belong to it and subtly contradicts it.

But what form does governmental practice take and what dynamics does it affect? It comprises an extremely animated and multifaceted domain, which ranges from Christian pastoral to reason of state and the police state, from the sciences of cameralism and mercantilism to those of physiocracy and political economy. The common denominator that holds these segments of knowledge together is the new object they address from a certain moment on: the population, which, along with security strategies, is the main topic of the 1978 course. But the important point, as far as Foucault's discourse is concerned, is that governmental practice arises from a source that differs from that of classical Greek and Roman political theory and generally conforms to the principle "the king reigns but does not govern." Found initially in Egypt, Assyria, and Mesopotamia, the metaphor of the shepherd who leads his flock, understood as a form of protection and care, finds its chosen place first in Judaism and then in Christian treatises, in a form that cannot be likened to sovereign power. At its core is a relationship, at once individualizing and totalizing, between command and obedience that is foreign to the classical tradition of rule of law and monopoly of power. In the pastoral metaphor, the impersonal command of the law is replaced by a circular relationship between the shepherd's prudent care of each individual sheep and the flock's absolute submission to his directives. Their obedience is exhaustive and permanent – something unthinkable in ancient Greece or Rome – independent of the rationality of command, and gauged by mutual trust between the shepherd and the flock he leads.

Once this form of control over minds and bodies was emancipated from the divine economy and secularized in biopolitical *dispositifs*, it became the government of humans. At a certain point this practice, which originated on a terrain extraneous to the specifically political, crossed paths with the state and "governmentalized" it. Foucault insists on this point, which is crucial to the organization of the new paradigm: society does not undergo "statalization"; it is the state that is governmentalized. It is as if what lay outside the state seeped inside it or, conversely, incorporated it, thereby diminishing its status of pivotal linchpin for political technologies to one of tool for them. Against any ontology of the state as the sole bearer of power,

> What we would have to show would be how, from the sixteenth century, a civil society, or rather, quite simply a governmentalized society organized something both fragile and obsessive that is called the state. But the state is only an episode in government, and it is not government that is an instrument of the state.[36]

A major turning point thus occurred in the genealogy of western power; it was made possible by an equally radical theoretical watershed. That which appears to be the subject – the state – becomes the predicate of a dynamic that precedes it and determines its very functioning. This reversal of priority between the state and the technologies of government created a contradiction that was destined to weigh on all western politics, in a form that is far from being exhausted. What we usually regard as the political institution par excellence, the state, originated inside a nonpolitical sphere that absorbed it into its own economic *dispositifs* and ended up depoliticizing it. More than a subject of politics, the state is simply the principle of intelligibility required to think a posteriori about a multiplicity of institutions that pre-exist it. From this point of view, the government should not be set in opposition to power. Government is simply the mode for exercising power in the form of the economy – as liberalism would theorize, in the most explicit manner. But the question Foucault leaves open concerns the effect of this heterogeneity. What does it mean to say that western politics lies on a non-political ground and incorporates the nonpolitical inside itself? What does this shift into the negative imply for the functioning of modern systems of government? And what outcome does it have for biopolitics, which is the paradigmatic matrix and at the same time the historical effect of all this?

5

The course that Foucault gave the following year, called expressly *The Birth of Biopolitics*, did not respond fully to these questions. Foucault himself admitted that he originally thought his lectures in 1978–1979 would tackle this topic, but he realized that, for them to do so, he would first have to examine the governmental regime that biopolitics serves: "only when we know what this governmental regime called liberalism was, will we be able to grasp what biopolitics is."[37] Contrary to what has been argued by those who see this detour as an about-face, or even as an alignment with liberal positions, Foucault did not betray his original aims; on the contrary, he twisted them around to create a path back to the immune paradigm. What brings the paradigm back, albeit indirectly, is the issue of the negative that arose in the preceding course. It refers now not just to the dissonance between politics and governmentality – that is, the impolitical character of governmental practice – but also to the activity of governing itself. Given this antinomy, for the government to function within the liberal regime, it must *not* govern – or it must not do so beyond a certain limit, as Foucault argues in a programmatic passage:

> The whole question of critical governmental reason will turn on how not to govern too much. The objection is no longer to the abuse of sovereignty but to excessive government. And it is by reference to excessive government, or at any rate to the delimitation of what would be excessive for a government, that it will be possible to gauge the rationality of governmental practice.[38]

According to the principle of immunization as defined so far, for the government to express itself in the best possible way, it must limit itself by activating a kind of internal brake. This explains the semantic importance of "not": "So, with political economy we enter an age whose principle could be this: A government is never sufficiently aware that it always risks governing too much, or, a government never knows too well how to govern just enough."[39] Of course, the political economy asserts the interests it represents, adhering thoroughly to its own social object – the naturality of economic dynamics – to the point that liberalism can be understood as a form of naturalism. But this very adhesion to the natural principles that regulate human conduct requires a downscaling of the government. If, in the police state or in the administrative state, "the king reigns but does not govern," when it comes to liberal reason, it must be added that the government does not govern either, unless it keeps itself under a minimum threshold: to govern means to govern as little as possible. Foucault emphasizes the essential opposition between political sovereignty and economic government. "There is no sovereign in economics. There is no economic sovereign."[40] The economy snatches away from the sovereign – from the law and from politics, that is – what gradually becomes the epicenter of life in the biopolitical era: the relationship between people founded on their interests. From this standpoint, "the science of political economy" appears to be a contradiction in terms. Just as there can be no government of the economy, economics cannot make itself the science of government: the presence of one inhibits the presence of the other.

But the immunitarian reversion that Foucault impresses on his object of investigation does not stop at government activity. It impacts the concept essential to liberalism, that is, freedom itself. He starts by saying that there are two concepts and two genealogies of freedom: one, stemming from the French Revolution, is conceived of as an exercise of fundamental rights; the other, radical and British, is conceived of as the independence of the governed from their governors. These strands are not irreconcilable, of course, but they are noticeably heterogeneous. Although for some time the axioms of human rights were historically expressed through utilitarian calculations, at a certain point utilitarian reason predominated, marginalizing the other face of liberty. Just as happened to government practice, freedom came into contradiction with itself, ultimately negating its most powerful meaning. But there is more to be said. Even inside the liberal interpretation that gradually won out, there emerged an autoimmunization movement that made the production of freedom contingent on its negation. As is typical of the immune *dispositif*, limitation is the negative repercussion of an excess. Liberalism does not limit itself to defending given freedoms – it produces them, in the sense that, to function, it must extend them everywhere, from the market to trade and opinion. But to create them it must also organize them, protecting them from any dangers that may threaten them. A fracture thus forms in the heart of freedom and pushes toward its logically opposite dimension of security, giving rise to "an always different and mobile problematic relationship between the production of freedom and that which in the production of freedom risks limiting and destroying it."[41]

On the basis of the growing demand for security that pervades the liberal regime, the collective interest must be defended from the dangers posed by individual interests, but also vice versa. Society must be defended from individuals and individuals from society. This leads to a vicious circle between danger and security that increases both, in direct proportion with each other: the larger the perception of risk, the greater the need for security. Individuals are stimulated to "live dangerously," to load their lives with dangers, which exponentially increases the need for control, in contrast to the freedoms that liberalism aims to protect. Security strategies are the condition and, simultaneously, the reverse of freedom, their driving force and counterweight. A genuine immunitarian circuit emerges between security and danger, culminating in Bentham's Panopticon – a prison model for continuous surveillance and the main figure of liberal government. "This is, if you like, the ambiguity of all the devices which could be called 'liberogenic,' that is to say, devices intended to produce freedom which potentially risk producing exactly the opposite."[42] This internal contradiction is allied with the fact that, in order to combat its historical adversaries – fascism, communism, and social democracy – liberalism adopts defense methods that compromise the free development of society. Similarly, in a continual reversal of perspectives, even criticisms of liberalism fall within its framework; they, too, arise from the need to combine freedom and security. For example, Keynesian policies such as the New Deal and Welfare come into existence to guarantee the freedom of workers against the risk of unemployment. But the only way to implement them is by limiting individual freedoms; hence the crisis of the liberal system in the 1930s that, after World War II, led to the neoliberal revision of liberalism in Germany and the United States.[43]

In Foucault's eyes, from this vantage point every economic planning idea appears destined sooner or later to fail. This is not to say that he subscribes to the liberal view; on the contrary, he identifies all its limitations inherent in the immunitarian turn. But he does believe that countering it requires a response on an equal footing, without retreating to positions superseded by history. The missing element is a notion of political government adequate to the predominance of economic interests. Limiting the sovereign's powers is not enough for *Homo oeconomicus*, who explodes the sovereign's blind spot: that is, the inability to encompass in a single view a society no longer associated with a shared horizon. The very idea that the government is able to fulfil a general interest – in other words, to politically mediate individual interests – turns out to be essentially utopian. Every government that sets itself this objective creates a counterproductive effect that betrays its own intentions. Adam Smith's theory of the "invisible hand," in other words, of the spontaneous harmony between diverging interests, makes any sovereign operation meaningless. From the perspective of physiocracy – which demands that "the sovereign will have to pass from political activity to theoretical passivity in relation to the economic process"[44] – sovereign intervention is still possible, although already scaled down; but when economic subjectivity exceeds juridical subjectivity, it is forced to retreat completely. The law, like politics, no longer appears capable of resolving the issue of how to govern a society directed by the economy. Its resolution lies neither in market autonomy nor in the old figure of the social contract, which imagines transcending the state of nature.

Foucault's answer is that the only way of revitalizing a governmentality threatened by extinction, of putting the government machinery back into motion, is to secure it a new object, that of "civil society." Like all the concepts that Foucault examines – madness, sexuality, population – civil society should not be seen as a natural given but as the effect of a technology set up by the economic regime itself. By comparison with the civil society that Locke or otherwise Hegel write about, that of Ferguson and Smith, to which Foucault refers, is the concrete globality within which *homines oeconomici* move about. Its role is to create a spontaneous synthesis of individuals through "disinterested interests" – generated, that is, through sharing, sympathy, and benevolence rather than through a selfish drive. But in this case, too, the resulting sociality is undermined by its own content, which still consists in economic competition. Once again, the political government of the economy proves to be impossible, because it is contradicted by its own substance. The economic society is united by its own insuperable division. It gets united by separating and associates by dissociating: "The economic bond . . . constantly tends to undo what the spontaneous bond of civil society has joined together . . . In other words, the economic bond arises within civil society, is only possible through [civil society], and in a way strengthens it, but in another way it undoes it."[45]

The immune mechanism that binds the economy and the government in an aporetic form reappears from this angle, too, revealing itself to be at odds with the community, to which it is nevertheless intrinsic. Not even in this interpretation, then – in a course dedicated to its birth – does biopolitics find an affirmative form. Articulated on the immune paradigm, it shares in its essential ambivalence. As soon as it is rejoined with the economic government it serves, it can define it only negatively – as a practice that is socially necessary but impracticable in political form.

6

How can we break the negative cycle of liberal biopolitics? Or, to put it differently, how can we open a new site to construct an affirmative biopolitics? To answer this question, we need to take a step forward – or sideways – from Foucault's discourse. Once we acknowledge the incongruous character of the criticisms launched against him – the generic nature of the biopolitical paradigm, its lack of historical depth, and its metaphysical tone – something more (or different) must be added, namely about his less than adequate notion of the relationship between politics and life. It can hardly be said that these two words are seamlessly integrated in his conceptual apparatus. The impression remains that, instead of being fused in a single semantic block, they were developed separately and then only later melded together into the concept of biopolitics. This may be the reason why Foucault redefines it in some way, although without abandoning it, or generalizes it in the not altogether analogous concept of governmentality. Then again, without this structural dissonance, it would be difficult to understand why the notion he invented was then pulled apart by other interpreters in such a way as to have one of the poles absolutized to the detriment of the other – by either unduly superimposing power on top of life or – conversely – by granting life a constituent power independent of the political condition.

Clearly this does not mean that the two polarities of biopolitics cannot coincide or pass through each other in a linear fashion. As also Thomas Lemke argues,[46] they always meet up in a provisional relationship, which changes depending on the phase and the context. But the establishment of their boundary line is not naturally given; it too is the effect of political action within a particular historical framework. While it is clear that the healthcare biopolitics of the late eighteenth century is different from the securitarian biopolitics of the nineteenth, it is a far cry from Nazi biopower. To maintain that a single thread connects completely heterogeneous episodes – or even that the sovereign relationship between power and life dates to the dawn of western history and extends into our time – is misguided when it comes to an intensely historical approach such as Foucault's. If any critical observation can be made, it is that his own theory must be historicized, something he was obviously not in a position to do from where he sat. As we have seen, rereading his three great courses on biopolitics makes apparent the thematic and lexical distance that separates the first one, on conflict, from the other two, focused as they are on the concept of government. A binary – and oppositional – interpretation of society gives way to a reading unified by the increasingly fluid relationship between the governors and the governed. It is as if the two perspectives, both of which describe the biopolitical regime but capture it at different levels of historical depth, were unable to find a point of connection – or a more balanced arrangement – between government and conflict. For just as war between peoples, at least within each of them, is itself a governmental strategy, so the government of the living remains traversed by a profound disagreement between social segments that are too unequal to merge into a single body politic.

Only by recognizing this implication can we account for a perverse effect of the biopolitical paradigm: its reversal in a thanapolitical direction, especially in the first half of the twentieth century. Certainly, in this case too we must be cautious about generalizations and guard against lumping together situations and contexts that are incomparable, such as the Nazi extermination camps and the exclusions, or even the violence, of today's biopolitical regimes. Nicolas Rose has rightly underscored the distance that separates the eugenics of the 1930s from contemporary genetics or genomics.[47] To avoid a purely rhetorical formulation, we must distinguish the theory of eugenics – which, from Galton on, targeted populations, understood as closed societies territorialized inside a national perimeter and often identified with a race – from later genomic research aimed at treating single individuals affected or threatened by hereditary diseases. The former proclaims the racial superiority of certain peoples and ultimately excludes or eliminates those whom it believes contaminate its purity, whereas the latter has primarily therapeutic aims, intended for single individuals. A top-down, state-led eugenics is contrasted with a ground-up science tailored to individuals. This does not preclude a subtle thread of continuity that runs between the two modes of intervention into biological life, namely the assumption that it is possible to operate on human nature in order to improve it. Not only did the eugenics of the first half of the nineteenth century leave more than a few traces in our current public health system, but also a clear disproportion exists between nations that possess the resources to fund this type of research and nations that are nowhere near having this capacity. It could be said that out of the old racism there arose a new de facto racism, which links some endemic diseases to particular ethnic groups, and these are condemned by their social conditions to become carriers. One need only measure the difference between the biomedical resources of wealthy nations, which possess them in abundance, and those of underdeveloped peoples: only a minimal, absolutely insufficient portion is destined to the majority of the world's population. A few hundred dollars a month would be enough to save a large number of children who are otherwise condemned to certain death. As Rose reminds us, millions of lives continue to be cut short by factors such as poverty and lack of food, water, hygiene, and medicines. What is missing, more than individual efforts, is institutions capable of permanently reversing this catastrophic trend. When we count the frightening number of people who have fallen victim to malnutrition, disease, and war and compare it to numbers in socially protected groups, it is difficult not to think of the irremediable division Primo Levi described between the drowned and the saved, or of the biopolitical contrast between those who are kept alive and those who are left to die.

This dramatic dialectic is precisely what Foucault sketched out in the mid-1970s; but it faded away, or even disappeared altogether, in the courses he gave toward the end of the decade. Didier Fassin, perhaps overly harsh in his judgment, sees this withdrawal as a blind spot in Foucault's perspective: in his view, biopolitics "does not correspond to what the etymology of the word suggests. It does not fall under politics as much as under govern-mentality, and its subject is the population rather than life: biopolitics is not a politics of life, it is a governing of populations."[48] By emphasizing the various technologies of government rather than their actual effect, biopolitics avoids examining the way politics concretely treats the lives of individuals, putting its focus instead on the *dispositifs*. For this reason, Foucault's biopolitics need to be translated into a politics of life – or, better yet, of lives – given the vast difference created by their unequal treatment. Fassin notes a clear distinction between such a politics of life and the widespread sacralization of biological life, turned into an absolute value to which all others must be sacrificed. This distinction becomes central to his work, which is focused on identifying inequalities that cut across the experience of human beings along precise social, ethnic, and cultural boundaries. More specifically, Fassin identifies an episte-mological threshold, located at the beginning of the 1990s, beyond which the value of sociopolitical life gradually diminished to the benefit of natural biological life. This choice for simple survival over socially defined forms of life can be found in French immigration policies as well as in South African debates on the distribution of antiretroviral drugs, the two case studies he analyzes. In both contexts, there is a clash between two different ethics: one assigns absolute priority to the preservation of human life, while the other takes into account more complex sociopolitical issues. According to Rose, the increasingly stark predominance of the former over the latter marks the emergence of a kind of biolegitimacy, that is, the emergence of the primacy of the *conservatio vitae* mandate over and above any other consideration. Just like in France – where the risk to migrants' biological life appears more important than their request for political asylum – in South Africa, too, protection from AIDS takes precedence over the fight against social inequality.

As we shall see in what follows, this evaluation remains highly controversial, especially during the time of the pandemic. The fact remains that today "physical and biological life has a material presence that imposes itself on all and sundry, with a visibility that social and political life lacks";[49] hence the critical need to counter the ethical slide toward a biolegitimacy that takes space away from political initiative. This critical awareness, says Fassin, is missing from Foucault. In the circular relationship between power and resistance, the word "inequality" ends up disappearing from his vocabulary. At issue is not what Foucault said but rather what he failed to say. The biopolitics he theorized captured a problem crucial to our time but, until his discourse is updated to reflect current sociopolitical dynamics, it will not help to resolve it.

7

The other piece missing from Foucault's biopolitics relates to the problem area of institutions. It is not that he neglected it, in his work or in his personal life, because in a certain sense one could even say that he did nothing else. Hospitals, prisons, orphanages, asylums for the insane, and monasteries were always central to his interests, both in his research and in his politics. Nevertheless, from the start, his look at institutions was not direct but mediated through the power relations that produce and exceed them – first, because institutions are located at the crossroads of the various lexicons of administration, family, healthcare, education, and sexuality – which implement one another; and, second, because they are traversed by tensions and conflicts that modify their profile over time according to the shifting balances of power. From this point of view, both spatially and temporally, no institution coincides permanently with itself, or at least with what it claims to be. This applies first to the institution that appears to head all the others: the state, structured in a series of apparatuses understood as "relais-multipliers of power within a society in which the state structure remains the condition for the functioning of these institutions."[50] But, even though the state fulfills this role, it cannot be said to represent faithfully the society from which it emerges. By concentrating attention on itself, eventually it distracts society from the tactical, contingent relations that underlie it and need to be reconstructed in their specificity. Foucault is quick to express his misgivings about this:

> Now I no longer think that the institution is [a] very satisfactory notion. It seems to me that it harbors a number of dangers, because as soon as we talk about institutions we are basically talking about both individuals and the group, we take the individual, the group, and the rules which govern them as given, and as a result we can throw in all the psychological or sociological discourses.[51]

The discourse that institutions, taken as an object of direct study, risk legitimizing most of all is the juridical discourse, which Foucault always viewed with some suspicion. Institutions do not express particular norms, because they are the result of technologies whose effects are different from the declared aims. For example, instead of fighting crime, incarceration ends up reproducing it, exactly the way psychiatric hospitals often aggravate the diseases they are supposed to cure. For this reason, Foucault's interest does not lie so much in the purpose an institution declares as in the social control function it performs in political regimes. In the final analysis, despite the heterogeneity of the languages involved in institutions, their role remains coercive – organized according to the prison model, of which Bentham's Panopticon remains the unparalleled archetype. While not necessarily "total," like those analyzed by Erving Goffman in *Asylums*,[52] they are associated by Foucault with the notion of "sequestering." Despite their declarations and even their intentions, institutions perform a role that is substantially repressive, or at least conservative. Consequently they cannot be reformed – not because they are fixed in time, but because even the reformist logic is organic to their preservation. Even the resistance that institutions provoke proves useful to what is being contested and ends up reinforcing it. Since institutions do not exist as such, except as terminals of underlying powers, they appear to be unassailable. Considered unreformable, they can only be bypassed, or de-instituted, by reversing the way they were instituted historically.

But this is not Foucault's final, or only, word on institutions. In the course examined earlier, on the birth of biopolitics, he opens a partly new discourse on institutions, referring more to instituent power than to the instituted. In his lecture of February 21, 1979, on German ordoliberalism, Foucault brings new insights into the role of the law; more specifically, into the role of the juridical institution in a market-regulated society. Starting from Luis Rougier's talk at the 1939 Walter Lippmann conference, Foucault argues that the juridical phenomenon does not reside in the superstructure but "[t]he juridical gives form to the economic, and the economic would not be what it is without the juridical."[53] Thus, instead of employing the old dichotomy between economic infrastructure and legal superstructure, one should speak of an economic–legal order – what Walter Eucken calls "system." It certainly refers to economic processes, but processes that would not have occurred outside an institutional framework of shared rules. This has a more general significance – and, as

Foucault points out, a political stake – which concerns the reality of capitalism, whose history has an economic–institutional character.

But Foucault does not stop at this definition: he brings up another side of the issue, which he himself calls "legal interventionism." This phenomenon is not only different from economic interventionism, which is criticized in ordoliberal logic, but also ultimately replaces it:

> The consequence of this is no economic interventionism, or a minimum of economic interventionism, and maximum legal interventionism. . . . For Eucken, the historians' unconscious is not the economic but the institutional; or rather, the institutional is not so much the historians' unconscious as the economists' unconscious.[54]

Let us take note: this is not just about retroactively legitimizing the given economic order but also about changing it through a set of institutional innovations that recall the system of government called Rechtsstaat in Germany and rule of law in the United Kingdom. Here, too, we need to be clear. In Foucault's interpretation of ordoliberalism, rule of law is not simply the positive alternative to despotism and to a police state, one in which acts of public power can be enacted only within the laws that limit it. It is also a system "in which every citizen has the concrete, institutionalized, and effective possibility of recourse against the public authorities."[55] This means that it is not limited to ensuring that public behavior complies with the law; it also provides for judicial bodies from outside the legislative branch that arbitrate relations between citizens and public powers in cases of dispute. This guarantees that power is limited, but it also protects the possibility to resist it: "the rule of law is a state in which citizens can appeal to ordinary justice against the public authorities."[56]

To fulfil this need, it is not enough to combine different judicial bodies to balance public and private powers. What Foucault is referring to is an intervention into economic processes through already established institutional bodies and also through new institutions. The particular policies that German ordoliberalism criticized in favor of the self-development of economic activity, including the American New Deal and British planning, have no importance now. What matters at a paradigmatic level is his objection to the idea that capitalism has definitively stabilized and the idea that follows from this, of possibly changing capitalism through the interventions of a power that can well be defined as instituent:

> So, first of all, an essential Capitalism (*le* capitalisme), with its logic, contradictions, and impasses[,] does not exist. Second, it now becomes perfectly possible to invent or devise a capitalism different from the first, different from the capitalism we have known, and whose essential principle would be a reorganization of the institutional framework in terms of the rule of law.[57]

This, adds Foucault, implies a renewal not only of the legal sphere but also of the judicial sphere, which, instead of being confined to simply applying the law, will assume an active role commensurate with the desired change: a judicial interventionism performed by existing institutions, but also by new institutions designed to put a true social interventionism into action.[58]

The fact that Foucault talks about all this during his course on the birth of biopolitics does not indicate a sudden change of direction but rather the insight, albeit left undeveloped and dormant, that an affirmative biopolitics must pass by way of a new discourse on instituent power.[59] This is not an easy task, for several reasons. First, because of the heterogeneity of the two conceptual lexicons; and, second, because of what has long appeared to be a clash of principles that is difficult to surmount. If Weberian institutional formalism was founded far from the horizon of life, biopolitics appeared to connect life and politics in a direct relationship, free from institutional mediations. In reality, both these perspectives have proven to be, if not false, then certainly unproductive, laying out paths that lead to no political end. Just as a formalistic institutionalism, external to vital dynamics, is locked in a self-referential orbit destined to be soon depleted, so an unmediated biopolitics, crushed into the bareness of a formless life, loses any political effectiveness. Both paradigms should go in the opposite direction. The call to institutions must be rescued from the conservative semantics of the ancient *institutio* and restored to the dynamics of the instituent movement; similarly, biopolitics must be freed from a biologistic approach and fully historicized – as Foucault did with it from the outset. In both cases, we are dealing with reconstructing the broken link between life and institutions. While institutions must be understood as living organisms destined to be born, grow, and eventually perish in favor of others, human life must be reconnected to the form that has distinguished it from the beginning. Life must be understood as something that goes beyond simple biological matter, something that, for that very reason, can define itself as a "form of life." Only in this way will biopolitics and institutions find the affirmative drive that gives a political value to our lives.

4

Philosophies of Immunity

1

The relationship between immunology and philosophy has long been solidified, as witnessed by the ever-growing number of studies on the subject.[1] Actually, it would be quite odd if a discipline like immunology, which revolves around concepts of identity and otherness, the proper and the common, preservation and evolution, did not appeal to writers and texts of philosophy. And in fact references to Plato and Aristotle, Locke and Leibniz, James and Husserl – not to mention Darwin, Nietzsche, and Foucault – abound in discussions between historians and theorists of biological immunity. But, just as immunologists call on philosophy, so philosophers put the immune paradigm to use. From their angle, the matter at hand is not thinking about immunology philosophically, but looking at philosophy from the perspective of immunological science. What makes this possible is not just the epistemological importance of the concept of immunity as it pertains to the cognitive sciences but also its ontological importance. Since community – understood as the constitutive relationship between human beings – has become an essential theme of contemporary philosophical reflection, it is natural that its reverse side – immunity – should receive the same interest, not simply as one topic among others but as the interpretive paradigm of our modern age, which has watched its centrality grow.

When we talk about the incidence of immune procedures, the idea is certainly not to circumscribe their presence to modernity alone, however. The need for immunization characterizes all forms of civilization, past and present, seeing that without some sort of immune system none of them would have been able to survive the disintegrative force of internal and external conflicts. In this vein, as we will see, the label "civilization" can be understood as a noble name given by historians to the immunization process, which enabled humans to persist in time and to progress. This does not detract, however, from the more specific relationship that makes modernity not only *an* age of immunity but *the* age of immunization, because what was formerly a given – the need for protection – becomes a problem in the modern era, and therefore also a strategic necessity. This happened at the end of the Middle Ages, when humans lost the immune devices that religion afforded them and were forced to construct other, artificial apparatuses in their stead in order to defend themselves from the mounting risks that threatened them. It was as if humans were suddenly expelled from the cosmic order in which they had been placed by ancient and medieval thought and found themselves in a world devoid of any centrality, wandering in space, with no precise destination.

Among the most widespread interpretations of modernity – as a process of rationalization (Weber), of secularization (Löwith), and of self-legitimization (Blumenberg), all useful for establishing distinctive features – the one that recalls the immune paradigm most forcefully, in a conceptual lexicon that is clearly irreducible to others, appears in Heidegger's essay "Die Zeit des Weltbildes" ("The Age of the World Picture"). Its connection to immunity lies in the specificity that Heidegger attributes to modernity as an "age of the world picture," in the sense that it is the only age in which the world is represented in the modality of the image – but also in the sense he gives to the words "world" and "image" and to their relationship. Because the notion of world includes the dimension of historicity, he strips it of any equivalence with the notions of cosmos and nature. But, most importantly, the concept of image assumes a meaning distinct from that of copy, to indicate the representation of something by means of an idea that presupposes it. For Heidegger, this representational modality does not designate a neutral description of a being but rather the act of "setting it before," with the aim of capturing it in its objectivity and thus of putting it at our disposal. In this way, between humans and beings there arises a specific relationship, constitutive of both, which makes the former the "subject" of the latter and the latter the "object" posited by the former. In a nutshell, then, what we are to understand by "the age of the world picture" is the intimate connection established, in representation, between subject and object, in a way never experienced before.

From this standpoint, without wanting to assimilate vastly different semantics, one can trace in Heidegger's discourse at least one thread of meaning related to the concept of immunization. The bridge between the two paradigms – of immunization and representation – is the category of "securedness" (*sicherstellen*) present in Heidegger's essay; and this is both the result and the presupposition of the world's reduction to image, which is typical of modernity. Securing is the specific form of modern science, understood as an investigation characterized by the claim to exactness and certainty of results. From there on, securing becomes a modality characteristic of the kind of representing that makes the world an object at the disposal of a being understood to be a subject: "This objectification of beings is accomplished in a setting-before, a representing [*Vor-stellen*], aimed at bringing each being before it in such a way that the man who calculates can be sure – and that means certain – of the being."[2] This demand for assurance pervades modern humanity's entire cognitive universe. While the mandate of science is to transform truth into certainty, starting with Descartes metaphysics, too, conceives of beings as objects of representation and of truth as certainty of method.

What is the relationship between this reassuring verification and the immunitarian need for protection? Certainly the two are not identical, but the former constitutes the logical premise for the latter. Only when modern humanity has pinned its knowledge of the world on definite coordinates can it reassure itself about the world in metaphysical terms: "With the interpretation of man as *subiectum*, Descartes created the metaphysical presupposition for future anthropology of every kind and tendency."[3] Modifying Heidegger's conceptual language, we can say that what he defines as "metaphysics" is the immune screen via which *Dasein* escapes from its dependence on Being, by closing the opening in which *Dasein* is located and replacing it with a representational device. By presuming to be a subject before a represented object, *Dasein* effaces the ontological difference that permeates the object and precludes any question about its own original provenance. If, with a bold semantic slippage, we were to give Heidegger's *Mitdasein* the name of *communitas*, understood as the emptiness of identity that alters its members, we could define immunization as the attempt to fill up that emptiness, exonerating its members from the *munus* ("duty") they share with others. After all, *munus* also has the meaning of "gift," does it not? In that capacity, would it not have something to do with Being's "donating" itself to those who remain in relation to it?

Another link between the two lexicons can be found in the characterization of freedom that Heidegger attributes to Descartes and to the metaphysical tradition that starts from him. Like premodern freedom, modern freedom, too, is instituted in relation to a bond. But in modernity this bond is posited in human reason and in the certainty of its law rather than in the revealed truth: "Descartes' metaphysical task became the following: to create the metaphysical ground for the freeing of man to freedom considered as self-determination sure of itself."[4] In the modern world, to found freedom means to identify it, first and foremost, with the certainty that the subject acquires about itself – which reverberates in the certainty of the object placed before the subject. This is how a metaphysical circuit is created through which the subject's security is communicated to the object, and from there it returns to the subject. Descartes' method for certifying the existence of the *cogito*, once emancipated from the presupposition of God's existence, becomes the key that binds the entire edifice of modern science and metaphysics to a knowledge that is certain.

The "securing" (or, in our lexicon, "immunizing") character of representation, which was there from the beginning, becomes evident at this point. To represent means to present ourselves as subjective guarantors of what is set objectively before us. The act of calculating, in its turn, gives rise to self-security, since only scientific calculation guarantees the certainty of what is being investigated. Representation no longer alludes, as it did in the world of ancient Greece, to the unfolding of the horizon of *physis*; now it signifies a "grasping" and "apprehending," in the literal sense of appropriating what stands before one.

Heidegger captures the violent character of securing, describing it as a territory of aggression: "the laying hold and grasping of."[5] As in every immune process, the securing act of self-defense spills over into a preventative attack against anything that puts the self in danger. The Cartesian equation between *me cogitare* ("that I think") and *me esse* ("that I am") constitutes the fundamental formula of every self-securing calculation, trapping the entire space of experience in a bond from which nothing can escape. Thanks to this bond, humans feel secure about anything that may slip from their control, assigning themselves a privileged status among all beings. This intensely metaphysical move explains how humans can declare themselves to be the measure of all things – not as the just measure between extremes, but as the right to judge everything representable. Once humanity establishes itself as *subiectum*, that is, as the foundation of itself and of the objectivity counterposed to it, everything becomes fully available to it. Nothing can get past it or sneak up from behind it, since everything is "set before" and exposed to human "awareness." Humans are now the arbiters of their own subjectivity, which they can narrow or broaden at will, passing from the individual to the collective form, encompassing a "nation," a "people," or a "race."[6] Note that Heidegger's essay dates from 1938, when he had not yet stepped back definitively from Nazism. In a few powerful pages, without ever exiting his own conceptual language, Heidegger effectively outlines the modern genesis of the immunization process, along with the dangers into which it risks precipitating modern humankind when it is freed from any common measure.

2

But on closer inspection it was really Nietzsche who inaugurated the modern immunization paradigm. Although he does not explicitly elaborate on the concept, he runs through its entire phenomenology – from its beginnings to its development, up to the limit point at which it flips over into its opposite. All the concepts he uses turn out to be riddled with it and thus revealed in their internal contradiction, starting from the most important one: "life." Because life is posited before every other experience, it expresses an immune demand intended to save it from its own constitutive anxiety. Immunity, it could be said, is the self-defensive mode of a life that tends to go beyond itself – to gaze out onto the nothingness that surrounds it. That is because a life that is identical to the will to power and strives to assert itself beyond every limit needs a negative to rein in its impulse and keep it alive. This negative – corresponding to the need for immunity – is not original. It is a secondary device, indispensable for preventing the disintegrative consequences of life's instinct to affirm itself beyond itself: "Behold," [this secret life itself] said, "I am that *which must always overcome itself*."[7] But this is exactly what makes Zarathustra a sign of contradiction: if life must push itself out of itself in order to live to the utmost of its power, it risks losing itself as life and collapsing into its opposite – into what it is not. This is how absolute affirmation ends up negating itself, leading the living organism to death. Immunization is the only way to contain this risk of extinction, through a lesser negative, which is capable of keeping life alive.

Nietzsche recognizes the restrictive character of this preservation and criticizes the reactive form it takes against a will to live that is free from inhibiting restraints, as he notes in a passage about Spinoza: "The wish to preserve oneself is the symptom of a condition of distress, of a limitation of the really fundamental instinct of life which aims at *the expansion of power*."[8] Nietzsche's criticism extends to all modernity, understood specifically as the age of immunization. "The democratization of Europe, is, it seems, a link in the chain of those tremendous prophylactic measures which are the conception of modern times."[9] The first chains he calls into question are the logical categories that undergird modern philosophy: identity, cause, non-contradiction – not forgetting an idea of truth that is indistinguishable from falsehood because it is designed to protect us from the shattering of meaning that we experience. These are immunizing measures that provide humans with the means to orient their thoughts and guide their actions when they have lost all bearings. By creating meanings that would otherwise be absent, they help us build embankments to contain the bewilderment that would otherwise paralyze us.

Nietzsche's sledgehammer of critique falls just as heavily on political institutions, associated as they are with moral prescriptions and religious convictions – all aimed at mastering the fear that gives rise to the modern immune perspective. With absolute lucidity, Nietzsche grasps both aspects of this perspective: one is necessary for the defense of life, the other is against life. Although this fear is indispensable for experience, as is the concept of truth, it ends up obstructing life's energetic sources, just as legal and political institutions protect life and at the same time negate it. They protect it by sheltering it from its own excesses and negate it by hindering its free development. It is thus true that the state – which modern political philosophy puts at the base of the *conservatio vitae* injunction – "is a prudent institution for the protection of individuals against one another"; but "if it is completed and perfected too far it will in the end enfeeble the individual and, indeed, dissolve him – that is to say, thwart the original purpose of the state in the most thorough way possible."[10] Immunization at high doses inhibits the innovative dynamic, rendering sterile the organism it serves to protect.

Nietzsche's elaboration of the immune paradigm does not stop at identifying this contradiction, though. It also seeps into his lexicon, which from the beginning shows a tendency to assume biological, and especially medical tones. The immune remedy is like a medicine used to battle an incurable disease, because it coincides with the vital force itself: "the worst sickness of mankind originated in the way in which they have combated their sicknesses, and what seemed to cure has in the long run produced something worse than that which it was supposed to overcome."[11] Here he captures the contradictory character of the immune mechanism. When immunization reacts to the action of the ailment without being able to eliminate it, it remains subordinate and ends up expressing itself in the language of its adversary. In trying to negate the ill, or rather repudiate it, the immune *dispositif* speaks the same idiom that it seeks to contest. Playing in the field of the enemy it seeks to defeat, it ends up being defeated by it. Immunization replaces a fullness – the original evil

– with an emptiness, a strength with a weakness, a plus with a minus. This is how it weakens the strong but at the same time strengthens the weak. In medical language, the organism produces antigens to activate its own antibodies but, in doing so, risks succumbing to the poison it injects inside itself. This is exactly what the shepherd of souls does to his flock in the economy of salvation: "He brings with him, doubtless, salve and balsam; but before he can play the physician he must first wound; so, while he soothes the pain which the wound makes, *he at the same time poisons the wound*."[12] If the drug contains the same substance as the virus it seeks to subdue – as in the practice of vaccination – then it remains inside the disease's circle, amplifying its disruptive effects. Of course, for the vaccination to work, as we well know, it cannot go above a certain dose. But the problem raised by Nietzsche concerns the logic of the immune procedure. If life itself is sick, and humans along with it, then any drug intended to contain it has, like any poison, a taste of death.

The tip of Nietzsche's critical sword, once pointed at priests and saviors, now sinks into the body of modern civilization itself. The civilizing process, of which modernity is the provisional outcome, carries with it structurally contradictory consequences. On the one hand, it facilitates life, saving it from the lethal dangers that bear down on it. On the other hand, by this very action, it weakens it. This obsession with duration – with preservation – is precisely what impedes life's development, condemning it to never achieve fulfilment. By wanting to separate – as does modern ideology – the being and the becoming of the living body, it paralyzes life, which is always necessarily in a state of becoming: "What benefits the individual's *duration* could put him at a disadvantage when it comes to his force and splendour; what conserves the individual could hold him back and arrest his development."[13] Preservation is not synonymous with development. One is the contrary of the other. What drives modernity toward its nihilistic drift is its lack of understanding about this opposition – the presumption of "preserving" development without realizing that in this way it impedes it. When life limits itself to surviving, it negates itself: it surrenders itself to the very negation it seeks to control. Then again, even if the evil is not restrained by the immune apparatuses installed by modernity, it will spread all the same, brought to extremes by the blind flow of a life that knows no bounds.

All of Nietzsche's work expresses this drama, namely the impossibility of the dialectic that in Hegel could still draw its affirmation from a productive tension with the negative. That possibility is now excluded as a result of a fracture that seems to swallow up all mediation. Life cannot be curbed in its expansive impulse, nor can it be projected beyond its own barriers. It is in any case destined to destroy itself, either explosively or implosively, through strength or weakness, disease or medicine. The only chance possibly still open of saving the organism from disintegration is not to rescue it from disease but to take disease as it is – in its mobilizing, innovative, productive aspect – without opposing to it a mythical idea of perfect health: "For there is no health as such, and all attempts to define a thing that way have been wretched failures"[14] – not only because it has never been clear what health, and therefore sickness, really is, but also because health and sickness are inseparable. Sickness is not the opposite of health – if anything, sickness is its reverse, its face in shadow. Or, better yet, its presupposition. One cannot exist without the other: "Finally, the great question would still remain whether we can really dispense with illness – even for the sake of our virtue – and whether our thirst for knowledge and self-knowledge in particular does not require the sick soul as much as the healthy."[15] This is why the ancient Greeks venerated disease as a god, as long as it was powerful. Health is not a good in itself; nor is it forever. It is only a good in itself if it is the beneficial transition between two states of illness. More than a possession, it is an acquisition, something "that one does not merely have but also acquires continually, and must acquire because one gives it up again and again, and must give it up."[16]

In a section in *Human, All Too Human*, Nietzsche takes his criticism of the immune paradigm even further, touching on the notion of *communitas*, against which *immunitas* stands out by contrast. The text is about a community united by equal conditions and by *munus*. Life is menaced not by an external danger but rather by the preventative action taken to protect it from risk; and in the end this action blocks its energy and innovative power. Although the community avoids the degeneration Nietzsche condemns in other, better known passages, it ends up blunting its self-generative potentiality and finishes in stasis. This time it is not the strongest individuals who provoke a beneficial wound to the whole community in order to avert this scenario, but the weakest, because they are the ones able to put themselves at risk: "It is precisely at this injured and weakened spot that the whole body is as it were *inoculated* with something new . . . Degenerate natures are of the highest significance wherever progress is to be effected."[17] Admittedly this is an isolated passage in the Nietzschean corpus, generally aimed at rejecting, even violently, any form of degeneration. But it holds particular importance insofar as it opens an original and unexpected insight – not into the negation of the immune paradigm, but into its possible convergence with *communitas*, understood in the most extreme sense: as an opening to its own alteration. From this point of view, contagion between different beings should not be avoided, because it is required as the excess from which the social body of the community and the individual body can be "ennobled": "Then, however, the educator has to inflict injuries upon him, or employ the injuries inflicted on him by fate, and when he has thus come to experience pain and distress something new and noble can be inoculated into the injured places."[18] What Nietzsche announces here, albeit in clear contrast with his work as a whole, is a vector of meaning with the capacity to deconstruct the immune paradigm from within, to the point of making it overlap with its common reverse.

3

The thinker who responded first and foremost to Nietzsche's immune reading of modernity, from another outpost of twentieth-century reflection, is Freud. If we read through all his sociocultural texts – from *Totem and Taboo* to *The Future of an Illusion* and *Civilization and Its Discontents* – we find the two cornerstones of Nietzsche's hermeneutics, communicated in a different lexical weave. On the one hand, there is the ambivalence of the modernization process, both protective and negative toward human life, which Freud extends to the entire civilization; on the other, he transcribes it into a medical language that is fully functional for the psychoanalytical lexicon. As for ambivalence, religion is identified early on as a primary and potent immune *dispositif* intended to protect humans from any anxiety related to their mortal destiny; unfortunately it has a doubly negative effect. In the first place, it drains value from earthly life. But, most importantly, by projecting life's continuation into an otherworldly realm, it creates an illusory image. Freud gives it a pathological characterization: this image is not just simple deception but rather the result of an infantile neurosis that affects the entire human race. While being careful not to establish an overly direct parallelism between the ontogenetic growth of the individual and the phylogenetic development of the human species, he does note a correspondence between them. Just as children ask their parents to protect them from the external world, so the masses turn to divine authority to soothe their uncontainable anxiety in the face of death.

Like all immune processes, this liberation from the fear of death comes at a rather high cost, though, which Freud interprets in terms of neurosis. Paternal protection requires several major sacrifices, both in the childhood of individuals and in that of humanity, namely renunciation of the immediate satisfaction of the erotic impulses and aggressive instincts that have always characterized individual and collective life. The repression or sublimation in higher activities entailed by this renunciation creates neurotic imbalances for both. Indeed, it can be said that at the base of the religious phenomenon is an exchange, only apparently advantageous for the individual, between two orders of neurosis: "[devout believers'] acceptance of the universal neurosis spares them the task of constructing a personal one."[19] The immune character of religion is redoubled in this case: religion is a protection, neurotic in its turn, from another kind of neurosis, which threatens all individuals. In the same way, for Nietzsche a human being is a sick animal that can heal itself only by contracting a more widespread disease, which affects the entire species. Since there is no way to avoid a certain dose of psychosis, if individuals want to save themselves from a violent death, their only option is to resign themselves to a more general form of psychosis, which they can at least share with their own kind. From this point of view, the other great master of immunization apart from Nietzsche is Hobbes, from whom Freud draws his inspiration. In Hobbes' world, too, humans accept the limited fear of the Leviathan state, to which they have surrendered their rights, in order to escape the uncontrolled dread of being killed by their own kind.

Civilization and Its Discontents enlarges this picture to include the immune mechanisms that "civilize" our lives, distancing them from the dangerous lives of our ancestors. Along with religion but more broadly, even the civilizing dynamic presents a double face, at once salvific and oppressive. As Freud answered Einstein in their correspondence on the question of "why war?," we owe to the civilizing process "the best of what we have become, as well as a good part of what we suffer from."[20] To dominate the hostile forces of nature and satisfy our primary needs, civilization creates a malaise proportional to the inhibition of erotic impulses and aggressive instincts. This applies equally to moral prescriptions and to civil laws, both of which are intended to prevent human beings from seeking the pleasure that is intrinsic to their nature. Here, too, Freud does not stray far from Nietzsche's program in *The Genealogy of Morals*. Like Nietzsche, he sees the elaboration of ethical imperatives as an enormous immune canopy meant to shelter us from the uncontrolled spread of reciprocal conflict; and, not unlike him, he finds in this negative protection something that damages human beings as much as it benefits them.

The threat that this mechanism holds for civilization comes from an immunization extended to the entire social life, in other words from the internalization of the same violence that we seek to avoid. Civilization is depicted as an enormous *katechon*, which combats evil not by excluding it but by incorporating it into its own procedures. This is what happens in the civilizing process: aggressive impulses toward others, rather than being eliminated, are introjected by individuals in such a way as to displace the struggle between opposites to inside their own psyches: "[The individual's] aggressiveness is introjected, internalized; it is, in point of fact, sent back to where it came from – that is, it is directed towards his own ego."[21] This dynamic – which Norbert Elias would pick up again in his writings on civilization[22] – is made possible through the formation of a superego inside the ego that overlooks it and exerts an aggression toward it equal to the aggression it would gladly exert on others. This instills in it an implacable sense of guilt. Made even more onerous by being internalized, this struggle fuels the tragic tension that runs throughout Freud's book. Unlike any preceding or later philosophy of progress, Freud's theory of civilization and immunization seems to touch in these pages on a point of unresolvable contradiction.

His path would appear to come to a dead end. On the one hand, every new pulsion increases the superego's severity and the punishment inflicted through the sense of guilt. On the other hand, every new renunciation – through repression or sublimation – increases the level of neurosis already implicit in all dynamics of modernization. Freud asks himself whether, "under the influence of cultural urges, some civilizations, or some epochs of civilization – possibly the whole of mankind – have become 'neurotic.'"[23] And he doubts that there are any therapies able to cure them. Without precluding the possibility that the principle of Eros may sooner or later prevail over its eternal enemy, such a hypothesis is barred by the fact that the aggressive impulse is not simply opposed to the erotic impulse; in reality the former inhabits the latter, just as the death principle inhabits the pleasure principle, as Freud states in a work where even the title places death "beyond" pleasure.

The problem regards both the relationship between individuals and that between individuals and the community. Both are subject to civilization's need for immunity. But immunity, as we have seen, only works by way of negation – it protects by including the evil that it seeks to prevent. When neutralized on one side, the evil tends to explode from the other. Moved from the community and placed inside the individual, from here it is brought back to the community, enormously enhanced; and the community becomes the battleground between Eros and Thanatos, between the drive for life and the drive for death: "This struggle," writes Freud in increasingly Nietzschean tones, "is what all life essentially consists of, and the evolution of civilization may therefore be simply described as the struggle for life of the human species."[24] In one passage in particular he touches on the most delicate point of the issue, when he expresses his conviction that, for a community to survive – that is, to immunize itself against the dangers of dissolution that menace it – it must resort to an openly sacrificial strategy, by attacking one of its parts for the good of the whole: "It is always possible to bind together a considerable number of people in love, so long as there are other people left over to receive the manifestations of their aggressiveness,"[25] he states, without failing to mention the endless European persecutions of the Jews.

The other text that provided the generative matrix for *Civilization and Its Discontents*, that is, *Totem and Taboo*, revolves around a sacrificial victim – the master father massacred by the brothers, who having been "driven out came together, killed and devoured their father and so made an end of the patriarchal horde."[26] The origin of civilization, of every civilization, harks back to this first event, still shrouded in mythical fog: the incorporation of the dead, or, more profoundly, of death itself. This incorporation alone can give life to civilization, since the brothers, united to the father through an ambivalent feeling of love and hate, rather than simply bringing him down, identify with him, first repenting of their own guilt and then embracing the same prohibitions that he imposed on them. In this way "[t]he dead father became stronger than the living one had been – for events took the course we often see them follow in human affairs to this day."[27] Civilization is born from this act – from a double negation: from the negation of the father and the negation of this negation, which initiates a sacrificial dynamic made of the same renunciations that we find in *Civilization and Its Discontents*.

> What had up to then been prevented by his actual existence was thenceforward prohibited by the sons themselves, in accordance with the psychological procedure so familiar to us in psychoanalysis under the name of "deferred obedience." They revoked their deed by forbidding the killing of the totem, the substitute for their father; and they renounced its fruits by resigning their claim to the women who had now been set free.[28]

4

The thinker who explicitly connects the sacrificial *dispositif* and the immune paradigm is René Girard. His perspective takes its cue, albeit critically, from Freud's book on totemism. Girard's approach reveals Freud's extraordinary acumen, but also an uncertainty that holds the psychoanalyst back from his own discovery. The truth of Freud's text, according to Girard, lies in the connection he reveals between the civilizing process and collective murder. Freud was the first person to realize that we must take seriously, more than ethnology and anthropology had ever done, a set of mythical stories with little in common except their agreement on the fact that human community is built on the sacrifice of one individual by the many. Freud was weighed down, however, by an assortment of presuppositions that lend a fantastic air to his thesis. He never developed his insight to its end, stopping on the threshold of something Girard claims to see in all its crudeness: namely that ritual murder, far from being unique, is actually repeated ad infinitum, and is the cornerstone for understanding the immune connection that intertwines community and sacrifice. Sacrificial violence is a protective instrument of the community against a violence that would otherwise erupt uncontrollably. But, to clear Freud's insight of its opacity, we need to take a second step, which moves the sacrificial dynamic outside the psychoanalytic domain. This is the conceptual move from Oedipal desire – directed at the maternal object – to a desire that Girard defines as "mimetic" because it is activated by imitating another person's desire, which is triggered in its turn by the desire of yet another. From times immemorial, this mimetic chain, destined to reproduce greater and greater violence, could be stopped, it seemed, only by sacrificing a single victim – an act that saved the community from ruin.

This assumption is what locked the entire history of humankind into a spiral of violence. It is not that humans worship violence in itself. On the contrary, they try to protect themselves from it by limiting it. But the only way they can do it is through another form of violence, less destructive than the first because it is concentrated on a single scapegoat:

> Nonviolence appears as the gratuitous gift of violence; and there is some truth in this equation, for men are only capable of reconciling their differences at the expense of a

third party. The best men can hope for in their quest for non-violence is the unanimity-minus-one of the surrogate victim.[29]

As we know, to seek protection from one evil by means of a lesser evil of the same nature is exactly what the immune procedure does, from which Girard draws out the entire sacrificial dialectic. The intersection of the sacrificial paradigm with the immunological paradigm is not simply procedural in nature, though. In addition to reproducing its logic, it re-creates its content, which consists of the same violence – likened to a malefic fluid that runs through the entire social body. Along the channel dug by mimetic desire, violence circulates undisturbed, spreading throughout the community. This flow, which threatens to engulf the community in an unstoppable wave, takes the form of an epidemic or pandemic contagion. The proximity between evil and disease is much better understood in mythological literature than it is in modern knowledge, which, in seeking to confine the practice of infection to the field of medicine, expels the sacred from reality, thereby losing any profound understanding of it.

A similarly far-reaching gaze signals the superiority of the great tragic and literary myths over the modern attempts to demythologize them; these, by pulling apart semantically proximate phenomena, lose sight of the myths' overarching meaning. There are even primitive societies in which a highly contagious disease such as smallpox has its own god. The sick are consecrated to it, isolated from the community, and watched over by an initiate, believed to be immunized through direct contact with the divinity. No wonder that some interpreters found a certain kinship between the idea of ritual impurity – from which people try to protect themselves – and modern microbial theories, even though their research in this direction was blocked by the prejudice that prophylactic protection lies uniquely in modern hygiene protocols. Only a sweeping gaze such as Girard's is able to grasp the essential link that ties together disease and violence in a more general immune logic. When we isolate medicine from the social and anthropological spheres, we remain blind to the undifferentiated circulation of ritual violence in its immunological function. On the contrary, "[t]he assimilation of contagious diseases and all forms of violence – the latter also regarded as contagious in nature – is based on a number of complementary inferences that combine to form a strikingly coherent picture."[30]

The classical text in which this proximity stands out most blatantly is Sophocles' *Oedipus Rex*. What unites the two kinds of violence, natural and historical, is the figure of the plague. It is "what remains of the sacrificial crisis when is has been emptied of all violence. The plague introduces us ahead of time into the atmosphere of microbial medicine in the modern world."[31] The themes of parricide and incest, on which modern critics have focused their attention, are simply diversions destined to obfuscate the primary scene of violence represented by the plague. It spreads in the city until it reaches paroxysm through the dissolution of all social ties. At a certain moment everyone is sick, except Oedipus. This is when the symbolic exchange between evil and sacrifice is triggered. The only way to stop the evil is by turning it against the sole being who appears to be immune from it, thereby protecting all the others. Only through this act can the city, disfigured by the plague, stitch its image back together and heal itself, recomposing itself through the killing of a scapegoat. But the *symbolon* – and thus the unification of the many – passes through a new division. The city reunites symbolically by splitting itself into two parts: everyone minus one in the first; and the sacrificial victim, alone, in the other. The sacrifice of the victim, contrary to the theological reading, is not offered up to anyone, except to the community itself, immunized by a single violent act that saves it from the circulation of the evil. Even when, in modern societies, the sacrificial logic is replaced by the legal system, it will not escape the immune paradigm. On the contrary, the legal system will bring it to perfection, shifting the objective from prevention to cure. Instead of trying in vain to prevent a vendetta, as prelegal societies do, the law monopolizes and rationalizes it, making it "a highly effective technique for the cure."[32] The punishment that it inflicts, although legitimate, is still isomorphic to the sacrificial logic: a single guilty party in place of all the others, who are declared innocent.

The correspondences that Girard identifies between the sacrificial dynamic and the immune *dispositif* are so exact that even he is surprised: "And what about the modern practice of immunization and inoculation? ... The patient's defenses, according to modern theory, must be reinforced so that he can repulse a microbiotic invasion by his own means."[33] Both the sacrificial and the immune *dispositifs* are always about expelling an intruder that threatens to destroy the human body or the body politic. "The physician inoculates the patient with a minute amount of the disease, just as, in the course of the rites, the community is injected with a minute amount of violence, enabling it to ward off an attack of full-fledged violence. The analogies abound."[34] Everything seems to correspond, from the booster shots needed for some vaccines to the possibility of provoking autoimmune diseases when an excess of vaccine material turns it against those it should protect: "'Booster shots,' for instance, correspond to the repetition of sacrificial rites. And of course, in all varieties of 'sacrificial' protection there is always the danger of a catastrophic inversion; a too virulent vaccine, a too powerful pharmakon, can promote the illness it was supposed to prevent."[35]

This risk of self-destruction signals the limit beyond which the sacrificial–immune dynamic can be taken no further. "The sacrifice," states Girard in the book that follows *Violence and the Sacred* and intends to reveal "things hidden since the foundation of the world," "is simply another act of violence, one that is added to a succession of others, but it is the final act of violence, its last word."[36] What comes after this last word? What begins when the curtain comes down on sacrifice? Who, or what, takes its place? To answer these questions, Girard makes an about-face: instead of looking toward the future of modern civilization, he turns to the past, to its Christian beginnings. With this disruptive move, he reverses the sacrificial logic into its opposite. While ancient mythological culture tends to justify the founding murder and erase all its traces, persuading us that the killers are innocent and the victim guilty, the Gospels go in the other direction, by witnessing Christ's innocence and his persecutors' guilt. The Passion is presented as a blatant injustice and Satan is blamed for initiating the history of violence by unleashing mimetic desire and introducing violence into history. But, by revealing this mechanism, the Gospels make it impossible to perpetuate sacrifice. Jesus's sacrifice is not the last, but in ripping the veil off its deadly logic, it pushes history out of its sacrificial cover, bringing to an end the immune syndrome that holds the world hostage: "Never has violence so insolently asserted its dual role of 'poison' and 'remedy' . . . And the only way of repelling the evil is by way of the evil itself."[37]

But if this is the last straw, if the immune mechanism is now running on empty or even turned against the body it is supposed to defend, then what else awaits us? Where should we be looking? What messenger is approaching us? One thing is clear: we can no longer count on violence to contain itself. For violence to dissipate at the end of a very long cycle, "there must be an ecological field that can absorb the damage done in the process. Nowadays, this field covers the entire planet . . . The environment can no longer absorb the violence humans can unleash."[38] Far from looking to the past, in these remarks Girard appears to be probing the future. Even his reference to the Book of Revelation seems to go in this direction – more as an opening to an unprecedented future than as a fulfillment of the ages. An apocalypse does not mean the end of the world but, on the contrary, the beginning of another:

To say that we are objectively in an apocalyptic situation is in no way to "preach the end of the world." It is to say that mankind has become, for the first time, capable of destroying itself . . . We can no longer count on sacrificial resources based on false religions to keep this violence at bay. We are reaching a degree of self-awareness and responsibility that was never attained by those who lived before us.[39]

5

Niklas Luhmann – not a philosopher, but a sociologist able to transcend the boundaries of his discipline – is the first author to explicitly theorize the application of the immune paradigm to the social reality. When he writes that "certain historical tendencies stand out, indicating that, since the early modern period, and especially since the eighteenth century, endeavours to secure a social immunology have intensified,"[40] he is talking about his own research topic. The immunization process begun in the early modern period has extended to all realms of experience, becoming the "grammar" of all modern society: "Like the temporal and fact dimensions, the social dimension can multiply contradictions and thus help to constitute the social immune system."[41] Of course, Luhmann is well aware that the organismic comparison between living systems and social systems cannot be carried beyond a certain threshold: living systems tend to guarantee the continuity of life, whereas social systems involve a reciprocal connection between actions. That said, what links them more than by analogy is their shared autopoietic model. In his second research phase – which culminates in *Social Systems* – Luhmann passes from a functionalist, binary-type conception, founded on the distinction between system and environment, to a self-referential conception that is circular in character. In the latter, the system's stability is no longer guaranteed by the capacity to reduce environmental complexity, but rather by the capacity to produce it internally in a manageable fashion. Any operation that includes what it designates is self-referential, or autopoietic: "A problem formulation's self-referential structure always becomes apparent if the problem formulation is applied to itself."[42]

This does not mean that the goal of systems is simple self-preservation. On the contrary, they presuppose the necessity of their own evolution, but in a way that does not put the unity of the whole at risk. This result can be attained only by establishing a productive relationship with the negative that inhabits all systems. Since systems require a high degree of instability to be able to react to themselves and to their environment, they reproduce themselves not by presupposing security but by governing insecurity. This is exactly what the immune logic does through the functional use of contradictions. Contradictions should not be understood as an evil but as alarm signals activated to warn the system about potentially unsustainable dangers. "They [contradictions] serve as alarm signals, which circulate within the system and can be activated under specific conditions. If one wishes to tie them down to something determinate, then it should be to this function. They serve as an immune system within the system."[43] They create uncertainty in a measured way, highlighting the "double contingency" mechanism at the base of open systems – it is not only our own uncertainty that must be considered but that of others as well. This means ensuring the resilience of the systemic structure in situations of inevitable change – not by restoring the status quo but by providing for a transformation that does not provoke a collapse.

The correspondences with the biological immune logic are striking. Just as a cellular memory is generated in a living organism that allows it to react immediately whenever some harmful event repeats itself, so in social systems a second perturbation is recognized, filtered, and eliminated automatically without the need for further analysis. The system reproduces itself by selecting novel elements that are compatible with its resilience; it separates them out from those that could undermine it. Like pain, argues

Luhmann, contradiction elicits a self-reaction even without a precise cognition about what is happening: "This is why one can invoke an immune system and coordinate the theory of contradictions with an immunology. Immune systems also operate without cognition, knowledge of the environment, or analysis of disturbing factors; they merely discriminate things as not belonging."[44]

The functional use of negation serves this purpose: "The system does not immunize itself *against the no* but *with the help of the no*; it does not protect itself *against changes* but *with the help of changes* . . . or, to put this in terms of an older distinction, it protects through negation against annihilation."[45] Contradiction negates every pretense of absolute prediction that comes from the system – everything is always possible, including what appears impossible. It can endure by making time an internal component, but only under certain conditions. Flashing like an alarm signal, contradiction warns the system about anything that threatens its duration, while at the same time ensuring communication between its components.

The need for communication should not be understood as an additional given but as the epicenter of a systemic logic that, in the final analysis, is identical to it. Over the course of Luhmann's work, after the concept of cause was replaced by that of function, although it did not disappear altogether, it was superseded in its turn by the concept of communication. Communication has the crucial role of creating relations between the various subsystems that make up the social system. But it has the even more important role of expressing its form. The social system is essentially communicative. It does nothing but communicate – with two provisos. First, it is not the subjects that are communicating, as in Habermas' theory of communicative action; and, second, the system communicates only inside its own limits – it does not communicate with the outside. Social communication "observes itself within its world and describes the limitation of its own competence. Communication never becomes self-transcending."[46] It translates the external into the internal, exactly the same way in which closure is the precondition of opening for the system. "The new insight postulates closure as a condition of openness."[47] This brings about a relationship between communication and immunization that goes well beyond the oppositional symmetry between *communitas* and *immunitas*, to reach a complete overlap. Communication is nothing but the form of immunization, while immunization is the content of communication.

But which subsystem enables this overlap, making it manifest at the same time? The answer is the law, as Luhmann states explicitly: "[The] law serves to continue communication by other means."[48] Let us not lose sight of the fact that Girard argues the same idea, but in a different form: for him, the law merely translates therapeutically the aggregating function that sacrificial violence performs in a preventative form. Then again, from the outset, legal semantics is one aspect of the concept of immunity, alongside and in relation to biological semantics. To grasp the peculiar way in which Luhmann understands the law, we must let go of the interpretation given to it by the traditions of positive and natural law. For Luhmann, the function of the law is not to distinguish between legitimate and illegitimate actions; nor is it to suppose or impose a given order. It exceeds the oppositional schema of lawful and unlawful on every side. After all, the declaration that everyone is equal before the law, a premise of modern law, is never completely averse to violence. It is true that the law serves to provide certainty regarding non-obvious behavioral expectations. But it does so by incorporating the conflictual tension created by this non-obviousness, with the difference that, while premodern law resolved conflicts preventatively, modern law itself produces them in a legally governable form: "Law does not serve to avoid conflicts. . . . it leads to immensely greater opportunities for conflict. It merely seeks to avoid the violent resolution of conflicts and to make suitable forms of communication available for every conflict."[49] Along these lines, Luhmann can conclude that the law "serves to continue communication by other means."[50]

The "other means" included in the communicative activity are evidently those of the immune process, understood as the content of communication. Here, too, we see the connection between the two sides of *immunitas* – the legal and the biological. Like the immune memory of living systems, that of the law, which is constituted from its own tradition, allows it to "even make decisions without cognition."[51] The number of legal cases introduced over time – later proclaimed law – serves to anticipate possible conflicts, deactivating their explosive charge through their communication. This is the precise difference between contradiction and conflict. For contradictions to become conflicts, certain expectations need to be communicated, along with the others' refusal to accept them. In this case, the concept of conflict is always related "to a communicated 'no' that answers the previous communication."[52] Therefore it is wrong to blame conflicts on failures of communication, as does for example Habermas. Communication is not something that can fail. It is the autopoietic process of social systems, independent of the cooperative or antagonistic character of the intersubjective relations. Since communication is identical to immunization, it is not a particular sphere inside systems: it is their very form. For as long as systems have existed, they existed by immunizing their communication and by communicating their immunization. The law is the expression of this operation, which serves community and immunity at the same time: "Conflicts are operationalized contradictions that have become communication. They enable the conditioning of immunizing events."[53] If this is true, the keystone for the resilience of social systems is the reproduction of conflicts intended to be communicated and immunized at the same time – immunized by their own communication: "A society must offer many as yet unused opportunities for conflict if it wants to reproduce its immune system."[54]

The immune paradigm finds one of its most powerful representations in these pages by Luhmann – so powerful that it incorporates even its own description. Nothing exemplifies what it itself presupposes more than Luhmann's theory: by that I mean the complete overlap of immunization and communication. In the case at hand, what gets communicated is the lack of any perspectival distance between the theory and its object – the impossibility of a critical sphere in a society that communicates nothing except the universality of immunization. In a passage of singular intensity, the German sociologist understands the final threshold to be overstepped and portrays immunization as the figure of the community to come:

> Despite all political boundaries that exist inside it, there is now only one world society: and this is because universal communication has been created, because we have become aware of the fact that there is a common world and everybody's experience is contemporaneous, because a common death has become possible.[55]

6

With Jacques Derrida, the immune paradigm passes through a new hermeneutic phase, illuminating not just its foreground but also its shadowy side – its autoimmune underbelly. This is the area the French philosopher focuses on, to the point of viewing it not as a possible collapse but as the inevitable outcome of the immunization process. Since the process impinges on all spheres of human experience, autoimmunity becomes the general modality through which life relates to itself while at the same time affirming and negating itself, affirming itself negatively. From this point of view – the productive use of the negative – Derrida's meaning of immunity incorporates and adapts to his own lexicon conceptual modules used by other interpreters, whom we have already examined – from Nietzsche to Girard, passing through Freud. In Nietzsche, life finds a source of health in sickness; similarly, Derrida connects life and death in such a tight knot that he expresses it as the lemma "life death."* Something similar can be said about Freud: Derrida revisits *Beyond the Pleasure Principle* with remarkable care, dwelling on the coexistence of the pleasure principle and the death drive. As for Girard's sacrificial paradigm, Derrida at least takes up its semantics, making self-immunization, that is, immunity toward oneself, "the sacrifice of sacrifice."[56]

But let us proceed in order. Although the term "self-immunity" appears rather late in Derrida's work – specifically, in his book on Marx – its antinomic profile can be recognized in concepts developed before that, such as life's differential auto-affection for itself.[57] For Derrida, life can relate to itself only through the other; or, more precisely, through its own other, which is to say, through the mortality that inhabits it from the beginning. This means that the living ego, by bringing the non-ego inside itself, is forced to "take the immune defenses apparently meant for the non-ego: the enemy, the opposite, the adversary and direct them at once *for itself and against itself.*"[58] From this standpoint, we can say that the autoimmune structure is the ontological mode, that is, the differential mode, of every form of life in relation to the life of others, but also in relation to death. As Derrida writes about Freud, "[t]hat which guards life remains within the domain [*mouvance*] of that which guards death."[59]

This is not to deny that autoimmunity manifests itself more intensely in a few distinctive areas, to which the author pays particular attention. The first of these is religion, to which he dedicates his 1995 essay "Faith and Knowledge." Starting from the medical definition, taken in its broadest sense, Derrida comes to recognize "a sort of general logic of autoimmunization,"[60] which in this case concerns the relationship between faith and knowledge and between religion and science. Starting from the first centuries of the

---

* An allusion to Jacques Derrida's title: *Life Death*, trans. by P.-A. Brault and M. Naas. Chicago, IL: University of Chicago Press, 2020.

Christian era, juridical immunity found a particular specialization in canon law, around the inviolability of asylum for those who took refuge inside churches. In this regard, Derrida recalls that Pope Urban VIII created the Sacra Congregatio Jurisdictionis et Immunitatis Ecclesiasticae, a congregation or commission of church immunity, to monitor tax and military service exemptions granted to certain individuals in derogation from common justice. But the most characteristic aspect of the autoimmune process is the strange alliance that, despite its declared opposition, today unites religion with technological capitalism. Not only are the most advanced instruments of military technology used in current religious wars; Christianity itself, with the pope at its head, operates with greater and greater ease in a digitalized cyberspace that makes telecast images the most efficient means of propaganda.

This alliance takes the ambiguous form of autoimmunity. On the one hand, religion tends to immunize itself from scientific rationality, to safeguard its original purity; but, on the other, it uses for its own purposes the same tools it apparently fights against. It is as if the immune process were divided into two divergent foci within the same ellipse, each of which reacts simultaneously against the other and against itself: "Religion today allies itself with tele-technoscience, to which it reacts with all its forces. . . . It conducts a terrible war against that which protects it only by threatening it, according to this double and contradictory structure: immunitary and autoimmunitary."[61] Indeed, it could be observed that the secularization process, with its demythologizing function, was born from the same Christianity against which it now operates, threatening to gut it. This is true of every force, which, as Nietzsche teaches us, grows only in confrontation with a counterforce that at the same time opposes and strengthens it – no differently from what antibodies do in the immune system. But what interests Derrida is not so much the immune logic itself as its autoimmune reversion, triggered by such an intense reaction that it turns against the body it is supposed to defend, destroying it. He believes that this happens in all cases: once the defense *dispositif* is put in motion, it cannot stop itself; sooner or later it brings about its own self-destruction. It is as if the immunization process can express itself only hyperbolically, negating what it affirms – the body's protection – and ending in self-disintegration.[62]

This is the catastrophic dynamic that Derrida recognizes in the tragic event that ushered in the new millennium: the terrorist attack on the Twin Towers in Manhattan. In that event he sees three interrelated and overlapping times or phases, in which the "terrifying but fatal logic of the *autoimmunity of the unscathed*"[63] is empowered out of all measure, until it reaches a climax. The first phase was the Cold War, which came to its fulfillment and final convulsion in the clash between the United States and the Soviet Union in Afghanistan. Out of this came the double suicide produced by the September 11 attack: the suicide of the Islamic attackers who crashed into the Twin Towers, but also the suicide of the country that hosted, trained, and armed them with its own airplanes and airports, on its own territory. The second phase, or the second time, of the autoimmune derangement involves a condition even worse than the Cold War: the use of chemical and bacteriological weapons and the uncontrolled spread of the nuclear arsenal, an even less manageable risk that has loomed in the West. What ensues from it is a trauma, or a mourning, that is even more profound than the effect of the Manhattan apocalypse because, instead of coming from an event in the past, it arrives from a future whose catastrophic dimension is unfathomable. The threat the West glimpses in the gash opened by the collapse of the Twin Towers is all the more frightening as it is indeterminate. The third phase of the autoimmune process, which now involves the entire planet, is the response of the United States and its allies to Islamic terrorism, a response destined to transform the conflict with the "axis of evil" into a suicidal war for those who conduct it. As in any blind reaction, those immune impulses "produce, invent and feed the very monstrosity they claim to overcome."[64]

Naturally, Derrida is careful to side with the West in his reconstruction, recognizing in fundamentalist terrorism a monster that "spreads death and unleashes self-destruction in a desperate (autoimmune) gesture that attacks the blood of its own body."[65] But what he insists on is the now globalized character of the autoimmune logic – shared by fundamentalist terrorism and its democratic adversary. We have already seen, after September 11, that American democracy, which had opened its gates to its enemies in democratic fashion, was led to contradict its own principles, accepting the battleground chosen by the opponent. But, as we have said, this autoimmune tendency, far from being linked to a tragic event, is made of the same stuff as democracy. Democracy is constitutively furrowed by a contradiction that undermines its stability, threatening to precipitate it into its opposite. Fascism and Nazism both came to power, we will recall, by exploiting the electoral mechanisms of democracy. Widely diverging between the unreconcilable principles of freedom and equality, democracy is challenged by the difficult attempt to represent the majority while at the same time protecting minorities. We have seen that in Algeria, when immunizing itself against its other, democracy immunized itself against itself. To protect itself, it abolished itself provisionally. Like all Derrida's concepts, autoimmunization, too, is undecidable: it is undecidable what should prevail in democracy: a constitutive openness to events or the defense of boundaries; a welcoming of all types of differences or discrimination against others. This is a double bind that cannot be turned into a dialectic, a double bind in which both choices can be seen as legitimate and illegitimate at the same time – even though they mutually exclude each other, according to the antinomic logic of an immunity that strikes against itself, destroying itself.

Nevertheless, this should not be construed as an absolute condemnation of the autoimmune principle. In Derrida's interpretation, the principle is not entirely negative – not because a double negation produces an affirmation in dialectics, but because the autoimmune collapse of immunity opens a space, empty at the moment, for something else, which lies on the side of community. For good reason, in "Faith and Knowledge" Derrida had already coined the word "co-immunity." It is true that the autoimmune logic haunts every community as its supreme risk and that there is no such thing as a community free from immune tension – and therefore not in contradiction with itself. But the opposite is equally true: every immunity, as it self-destructs, opens itself to its converse, community:

> community as *com-mon auto-immunity*: no community <is possible> that would not cultivate its own auto-immunity ... This self-contesting attestation keeps the auto-immune community alive, which is to say, open to something other and more than itself: the other, the future, death, freedom.[66]

By destroying its own protections – in other words, the very principle of the "proper" or the *autos* – autoimmunity reveals its vulnerability to the community, destabilizing any ambition of absoluteness that it may nourish. The fact that Derrida cannot say anything more about it or give a name to this otherness to come does not detract from the promise it carries, stamped as it is on a threshold that has yet to be crossed.

7

While the previous authors give a more or less sizable space to the semantics of immunology, Peter Sloterdijk inscribes his entire work within it. At least his fundamental trilogy on "spheres," which abounds in original formulations and implications, is an elaboration of a "general immunology." This is not to say that he does not share a set of presuppositions with his predecessors, especially Nietzsche and Heidegger, and, from a different point of view, Luhmann. From Nietzsche he borrows the idea that human consciousness itself is an immune structure designed to produce religious or metaphysical protections for humans, who are sick by nature. From Heidegger he draws the ontological story line, which he reworks in terms of space rather than time. Cast into an inhospitable world, human beings, who are by nature ecstatic, that is, turned toward the outside, feel the need to build spherical envelopes inside which they can protect themselves: "Living in spheres means creating the dimension in which humans can be contained. Spheres are immune-systemically effective space creations for ecstatic beings that are operated upon by the outside."[67] Lastly, like Luhmann, Sloterdijk sees the immune logic layered in systemic configurations that extend from biology to law, philosophy, technology, and architecture. From an architectural perspective, the spheres are heated psychosocial containers that from the origins of hominization ensure that humans have a shared space, sheltered from the threatening pressure of the outside. From the maternal womb to contemporary metropolises – through caves, houses, villages, cities, countries, and empires – in increasingly sophisticated forms, human beings merely replicate the same gesture of sheltering themselves from a destabilizing decentering that pushes them from the inside to the outside.

Once the general character of immunization is defined, the immune *dispositifs* must be differentiated according to their mode and development. Sloterdijk distinguishes three types, interrelated and overlapping in their functions. The first – at least from an evolutionist perspective, although they were the last to be discovered – are the automatic and irreflexive biological systems contained in our bodies. Over time, alongside them, to complement them, two other types formed, which were meant to compensate for public and private injuries: on the one hand, socio-immunological procedures, especially legal and political ones, through which humans regulate conflicts; on the other, symbolic, psycho-immunological practices through which they cope with the otherwise unbearable awareness of their own mortality. *Homo immunologicus*[68] stands at the intersection of these vectors, busily giving natural life a shared environment and a symbolic meaning. Of course, there is an epistemological leap from biology to society – from nature to culture – that should not be ignored. However, this does not detract from the fact that human beings have always occupied themselves with building joints and connections that are not just possible but necessary to their very survival. Humans are literally "pontifical" – designed to build immune bridges between what is inside them and what leads toward cultural, technical, and artistic horizons. "Whoever enters the gardens of the human condition encounters the powerful layers of orderly internal and external actions with an immune-systemic tendency above biological substrates."[69]

In addition to this synchronic distinction between immune systems there is another, diachronic distinction that relates to the different phases of the human journey from the inside to the outside, in the framework of an uninterrupted globalization. To begin with, it must be clarified that for Sloterdijk globalization cannot be reduced to the usual meaning of this word. What we see today is only the final, chaotic segment of something that has gone on for a very long time, having been segmented into three phases that form the subject of the three volumes of *Sphären* (*Spheres*). The first globalization, defined as "cosmic-Uranian," concerns a microspheric dimension composed of the binary unit of the primordial mother–child couple. When we exit the maternal womb and are faced with the challenges of the open, we strive to reproduce it culturally, in a womb of much larger dimensions: the celestial vault. Inside this space, as theorized by pre- and post-Platonic Greek philosophers, the Earth, enveloped in a cosmic mantle, occupies a central, privileged place that reconstitutes in macroscopic dimensions the same fetal condition. Like a fetus in the maternal womb of the placenta, ancient humans felt surrounded and protected by the concentric circles of the cosmos, inside a reassuring geometry that contained their anxiety to a controllable extent. Classical metaphysics, which culminated in Christian theology, was the philosophical transposition of this need for reassurance. From this point of view, religion represents the primitive and most powerful immune canopy of humanity, as it vaccinates finite beings with a fragment of the infinite. Humans join together in religion to overcome their fear of death through a sort of immune negotiation with the divinity.

The second globalization, which Sloterdijk defines as "terrestrial," originates in the explosion of the cohesive, centered universe into an infinity of splinters hurled in diverging directions. Suddenly, during the first centuries of the second millennium, the immune cosmic-Uranian structures fall apart, crumbling in contact with unprecedented events such as geographic discoveries. The Earth, no longer bathed by the warmth of the celestial mantles, loses its central, protected position at the heart of the universe. Already oriented toward the outside by their nature, humans find themselves besieged by monstrous exteriorities that wash them with the icy wind of the stars. Thus the ontologically *ek-static* being recognizes that it is exposed to waves of freezing cold, which the cosmos, now bottomless, can no longer temper. Immersed in a clearing with no bulwarks, modern-day humans have had to learn to exist like a kernel without a shell. From that moment on, they begin to look at the Earth as the only natural habitat they can occupy, while the sky is emptied of its gods. The Earth thus becomes the only object of globalization, transporting the immunization principle from a transcendental to an immanent dimension. No longer able to live *in* a globe – either womb-like or cosmic – human beings are forced to live *on* a globe, clinging to the terrestrial crust like shipwreck survivors. To be modern means to lose natural protections, and therefore to have to create other, artificial ones and confront the cold outside with the political techniques of climate warming – as in a sort of self-produced greenhouse effect that compensates for the celestial swaddling that has been snatched away. This is a crucial step in the history of immunization: "after the turn to the Copernican world, the sky as an immune system was suddenly useless. Modernity is characterized by the technical production of its immunities."[70]

The absolute novelty of the modern age lies in the fact that for the first time – with the disappearance of the "all-enveloping" ancient cosmos – humankind is forced to move about on a rounded body, lost in the universe, where even the atmosphere is conceived of as the innermost stratum of the outside rather than as the furthermost edge of the Earth. Humans are protected from their own conflicts primarily by political institutions, which culminate in nation states and their legal codes. But even more tied to the first globalization are geographic maps, which derive in their turn from intercontinental voyages. They spread the sphericity of the world onto a horizontal plane, supporting Heidegger's world grasped as picture, from which we began. And all this while the birth of insurance companies mothballs the theological safeguards of the previous periods. Navigators and cartographers are the heroes of modernity – even more so than philosophers. This is before Jules Verne and Herman Melville, Columbus and Magellan realize, from the deck of their ships, that the terranean continents do not contain the sea but the other way around – that it is the sea that surrounds the Earth. A long time must pass before "continental" philosophy adjusts to this reality, since, despite everything, neither Kant nor Hegel – nor even Heidegger, shut up inside his autochthonous jargon – manage to pull up the anchor of thought to gain the mobile space of the ocean, as do Tocqueville and Emerson. Husserl, too, for that matter, calls the Earth *Ur-arche* or *Ur-heimat*, seeking in it the foundation of western reason. In the competition between modern insurance techniques and the philosophical claims of certainty introduced by the Cartesian immunization of doubt, the winners are undeniably the insurers. It is as if to say: "Insurance defeats evidence,"[71] or even "Prayer is good, insurance is better."[72]

The generalization of insurance strategies is precisely what ushers in the third globalization: an "electronic" one this time, born from the ruins of the first two. Money – and, later, the flow of the financial economy – replaces ships in the increasingly rapid circumnavigation of the world. Rather than the beginning of a new age, this marks the end of the historical series of epochs, and therefore also the end of all philosophies of history, whether progressive or regressive. After all, the most authoritative modern philosophy of history – Hegel's, which claims to be universal – was nothing but European philosophy's self-representation, in a project to appropriate a world in which colonization was both the premise and the payoff. At the end of World War II, what collapsed with the Bretton Woods Agreement was not only the largest immune system of society but the very order of history. It was no longer possible to reconstruct the connection between space and identity that until then had given the globe a geopolitical structure. Not just the center but also the periphery went missing, in a sort of global de-ontologizing of borders. A nearly evaporating, polyspheric world, unstable and gelatinous, took the place of the ancient spheres and eviscerated them. "Foams" – a word that gives the third volume of *Spheres* its subtitle – replace globes and macrospheric political formations, from which individuals ungluc themselves, breaking off their relationship with the common horizon. Societies become aggregations composed of autonomous entities, connected by no more than their solitude – solitary subjects, who have become ego spheres or self-referential world-humans [*uomini-mondo*]. On this post-historical and post-spherical horizon, which intensifies disparities in living conditions, *immunitas* reveals itself to be the opposite of *communitas*, and not just etymologically. It expresses what is neither common nor able to be made common by any shared project. If all history has been nothing but a struggle between competing immune systems, never more than today have the immune benefits of some corresponded to the shortfalls of others.

This fulfillment of immunity – which seems to reverse once again into its autoimmune double – also constitutes the limit beyond which it is impossible to proceed. Immunization, having reached its final border, threatens to turn on itself, self-destructing. By now, it would seem, the die is cast, unless we initiate a drastic paradigm shift. This would involve radically rethinking the constitutive link between immunity and community on the basis of this realization, by building a single common immunity, a co-immunity meant to protect human beings – not some *from* others but some *with* and *for* others: "From there on, a protectionism of the whole becomes the directive of immunitary reason."[73] If this were possible, humanity would become a political concept, not an abstract ideal but a global immune design – something like a "co-immunism" to come:

> Although communism was a conglomeration of a few correct ideas and many wrong ones, its reasonable part – the understanding that shared life interests of the highest order can only be realized within a horizon of universal co-operative asceticisms – will have to assert itself anew sooner or later. It presses for a macrostructure of global immunizations: co-immunism.[74]

5
Pandemic Policies

1

The magnitude of the change triggered by the pandemic during the last two years can be measured by reading Patrick Zylberman's book *Microbial Storms: Public Health in the Transatlantic World*, published just a few years earlier, in 2013. It offers a well-documented analysis of the European and American policies adopted between the late twentieth and early twenty-first centuries to counter the risks of pandemics and of bioterrorist attacks. Two creative genres played a more than marginal role in these policies: catastrophe novels and films that prefigured apocalyptic events; and scenarios developed by intelligence services, especially American ones, to head off attacks or equally disastrous epidemic events. Both types are products of the imagination, but are in direct correspondence with reality. Based as they are on information obtained from government agencies, they in turn influence political strategies, thereby intensifying the self-protective syndrome that continued to mount in the United States and Europe at the close of the last century.

Zylberman's thesis, corroborated by a wide range of references, is that there is an objective disproportion between the perception of danger and the actual danger represented by terrorism and pandemics. Especially when it comes to pandemics, the author reports that the fear is overblown by comparison with the risk. His idea is that the available data are overly manipulated to raise the threat threshold artificially, so as to bolster the defensive apparatus in an irrational manner: "a terrifying panic attack is possible at any moment. Today health security is the object or the pretext of a spiralling lapse into fiction. Examples reported are exaggerated figures, analogies without base, scenarios of biological terror."[1]

In the oscillation between an openly novelistic fiction and one that claims to be realistic – that of the scenario plannings set up by the American administration – it is hard to know where fiction ends and reality begins. Thus, in an increasingly marked overlap between health security and national security, a "logic of the worst" begins to propagate, amplifying the microbiological threat. Although the principle of preparedness may be justified, Zylberman polemicizes against "the spokespersons of catastrophism, who collect under the same concept strategic, environmental, and health threats," with the paradoxical result of "prophesying a catastrophe that one hopes will not occur in order to prevent it from occurring."[2] The aim of this security strategy is to gather citizen consensus – in a sort of civil religion – without taking into account any ensuing effects that may be counterproductive at other levels: "all attention is usually drawn toward assessing the threat, without moving at all – or doing so very rarely – to evaluate the risks and the costs, the gains and the losses associated with a response to the threat."[3]

Of course, to avoid unleashing a risk equal to or greater than the one to be counteracted, we must not push the need for protection beyond a certain threshold. On this we can all agree: the boundary between a necessary immunization and an autoimmune disease must always be kept in sight. Nevertheless, in the face of a catastrophe that has proven to be as bad as, if not worse than, the fictional scenarios, one is struck by what a sensational rebuttal the current pandemic is to claims of over-preparedness. Everything that is considered a dangerous exaggeration in *Microbial Storms* – at least as far as the pandemic risk is concerned – appears today to be even understated, by comparison with what has actually happened. Of course, eight years ago neither the author nor anyone else could have imagined what 2020 would bring. But, for readers of Zylberman's book today, there remains the impression of a mistaken assessment of the relations between imagination and reality. Reality, rather than imagination, now seems unbelievable. This renders entirely realistic the anticipations made by those who had seen, a few decades before it happened, something absolutely excessive and yet – for that very reason – absolutely real. From this point of view, Zylberman's book is extremely interesting if looked at from an angle different from the author's. He describes as essentially "false," as the fruit of a paranoid imagination, what was soon to come true – even more so than in the most pessimistic predictions.

After the 1950s and 1960s, when progress in antibiotic medicine had instilled a general confidence about winning the battle against major infective epidemics, the eruption of AIDS in the early 1980s drastically diminished such illusions. Later on the appearance of Ebola in Africa gave rise to new worries, as it was accompanied by the return of malaria, yellow fever, diphtheria, and cholera in the most economically depressed areas of the world. Despite vaccines, infectious diseases remained firmly entrenched as the number one cause of mortality in the world. Suddenly it became clear that viruses do not disappear: they replicate and mutate uncontrollably. With the arrival of SARS during the same period, apprehensions swelled exponentially. From then on a dramatic perception of the relationship between health and the state, a perception inclined to equate the idea of "security" in health and politics, began to spread. As we have seen, this semantic linkage is the driving force behind an increasingly accelerated immunization in all realms of individual and collective experience. At the beginning of the new century, the September 11, 2001 terrorist strike, followed by the threat of anthrax and smallpox attacks, marked the most intense merging point of political and biological terror, opening the way to emergency politics, first in the United States and later in Europe. In 2003 a Forum of Emerging Infections, later called the Forum on Microbial Threats, was held at the National Academies of Sciences, Engineering, and Medicine in Washington, DC; a year later the Department of Homeland Security was established, combining national security and public health into a single organization. The threat of pandemic disasters assumed the same importance as a terrorist disaster, which was itself perceived primarily in terms of a biological attack. Thus the preventative defense strategy initiated earlier by Clinton became George W. Bush's preventative war against terror.

This alliance between political administration, scientific environment, and media system contributed to the fanning of fears. The resounding success of Richard Preston's *The Cobra Event*[4] – which tells the story of a contagious lethal virus unleashed by a terrorist group in the United States – had a powerful influence on American government policy and on Clinton in particular. The writer was invited to give a talk at the annual conference of the National Institute of Allergy and Infectious Diseases, alongside well-known physicians and scientists. During the same period, after years of research in epidemic-struck areas, the journalist Laurie Garret wrote, in 1994, *The Coming Plague: Newly Emerging Diseases in a World Out of Balance*, which predicted a new lethal pandemic, and then, in 2000, *Betrayal of Trust*, in which she foresaw the public health collapse whose effects we are experiencing today.[5] In the meantime the Homeland Security Council developed various scenarios – including the evocatively named "Dark Winter" and "Atlantic Storm" – that simulated terrorist attacks with biological material and countermeasures to combat them. These are media exercises, war games of a sort;[6] but they are capable of anticipating events that are dramatically present today: clashes between the federal government and individual states, difficulties and delays in stocking vaccines and masks, insufficient distribution to hospitals, exceptional derogations of constitutional freedoms, continual tracking of the number of infected people and the reproduction rate of the virus, individual and herd immunity, public disorder, and intervention by armed forces. In the light of what happened in reality, it would be difficult to find even one entry on this list that is exaggerated. Zylberman's assertion that American and European health policies were overly influenced by pessimistic scenarios would have to be reversed today: they were not influenced enough, causing the hecatombs we have all witnessed. How many human lives could have been saved, had we believed more in those predictions or imaginative speculations?

Incidentally, writers and directors were not the only ones to talk about it. In February 2006, in Boston, when the famous American virologist Anthony Fauci was retracing the events of the Spanish flu, he called for a turn from "moderate pandemic" to "severe pandemic," predicting 30 million hospitalizations and 7 million deaths worldwide. A year earlier, Michael T. Osterholm, professor at the Minnesota School of Public Health and director of the Center for Infectious Disease Research and Policy at the University of Minnesota, wrote an article in *Foreign Affairs* called "Preparing for the Next Pandemic," in which he imagined that a new pandemic – after the avian influenza – would cause a global crisis. While facing a dramatic shortage of vaccines, hospitals would be inundated by so many patients as to be unable to cope, since they lacked respirators and masks. The army would be mobilized to defend the inadequate supplies, while the economy would plunge into crisis, with a vertical rise in unemployment. Now that vaccination has become widespread – but only in the wealthy parts of the planet – the situation may seem better. But who could have imagined that not one of Osterholm's predictions would be wrong?

2

One of the most unexpected effects of the Covid-19 pandemic is that it has reshaped long-standing ethical and political dilemmas in a completely unprecedented way. The first of these dilemmas concerns the relationship between the values of life and freedom. As is well known, this topic runs through the entire western culture, from ancient Greek tragedy to twentieth-century philosophy. It comes up especially in Hegel's *Phenomenology*, in the master–slave dialectic: a "slave" is someone who gives up his or her freedom in order to preserve his or her life. But, during the pandemic, matters that traditionally pertained to individual choice demanded public policies for combatting the disease. To what point can the public authorities' protective action against the virus limit citizens' fundamental freedoms? This is the question that politicians and scientists, jurists and philosophers, and also citizens themselves have been asking. In other words, what relationship is there between the right to life and the right to freedom, both of which are fundamental, in a period that seems to put them at odds? This question – handled differently in different countries, partly on the basis of different constitutions – was at the heart of a debate carried out in Germany between the philosopher Jürgen Habermas and the professor of law Klaus Günther.[7] It took place after a disturbing declaration made by the president of the Bundestag, Wolfgang Schäube. It said: "The fundamental rights limit one another mutually. But if there is an absolute value in our basic law, this is people's freedom. This is inviolable. But it does not preclude the fact that we must die."[8]

Habermas takes a clear distance from Schaübe's words. His terse reaction is hardly surprising if we bear in mind

Germany's traumatic past and the fact that the German philosopher had always believed in the inviolability of human nature,[9] now menaced by new biotechnologies. Although the protection of life and respect for freedom are both constitutional principles, they are not equivalent. Even if they are kept in a necessary balance, one of the two must always prevail in the end. Admittedly, in the Basic Law (*Grundgesetz*) for Germany [the German Constitution], the protection of life, cited in the second article, is preceded by a reference to human dignity, asserted in the first article. But, since the reference to dignity was used in a discriminatory manner in Nazism, it cannot constitute a preliminary condition for the general protection of life. In any case, dignity of life can be judged only in the first person, by whoever is directly involved. Certainly, human life amounts to more than simple life and, to express itself in all its potentiality, implies what Aristotle called "the good life." But in a pandemic crisis such as the one we have lived through, the defense of every single life cannot be subordinated to the well-being of a large part of the citizenry. In short, when survival is at stake, the balancing between competing values cannot go on indefinitely. There is a point beyond which we must make up our minds and choose one, even to the detriment of the other. In the end, says Habermas, we must opt for the right to live, with respect to which all other rights, including the right to freedom, must take a step back – not least because life is the ontological premise, that is, the condition of existence, of every other right.

Without colliding head on with Habermas, Günther views the question in a substantially different way. For him, no right is in itself unlimited before the law – not even the right to life. To begin with, beyond the death penalty, countries effectively hold a lien on the lives not only of their enemies but also of their own citizens. This applies to other circumstances as well – for example a kidnapping, in which the police are allowed to shoot the kidnapper in order to free the victim. Obviously, to be able to put even a single life at risk for the benefit of another, or even for the benefit of an entire society, we must be sure that what we are doing is necessary – that there is no alternative. The other issue to be kept in mind is the profound change that has taken place since the document was drafted. When the right to life was introduced into the second article of the German Constitution, it was viewed as a safeguard clause against the state; today the relationship appears to be reversed. Instead of considering the state apparatus a potential threat to individual freedoms, we ask from it a guarantee that it prevent or reduce its citizens' risks of death. The state must defend its citizens' lives not only from aggressions of all types but also from disease, through adequate therapeutic assistance. As is obvious, no society can allocate all its resources to the healthcare system or view health as the only area for protection with respect to other citizen interests – starting with the right to freedom. The trick lies in distinguishing unavoidable protective procedures from others that are avoidable, before forcing people to forfeit their liberty. From this perspective, it would be wrong to oppose immunity to freedom unconditionally, given that immunity, if contained within reasonable limits, forms the space required to exercise freedom, which would otherwise be impeded by the virus's resurgence.

Although we will not arrive at a definitive response to this highly problematic question,[10] something can be added. Assuming that the right to life is the logical and historical premise to every other right, we must avoid forcing the opposition of principle between values that can and, within certain limits, must not only coexist but also be conceptualized in their original interconnectedness. To do this, instead of looking at them from an individual point of view, we must look at them from a perspective that embraces the whole community. Here again, to return to the central theme of this book, the bond that for so long has rigidly linked the immune paradigm to the legal sphere must be loosened. No right can be absolutized with respect to the common interest in which our individual fates are embedded. The right to freedom, if taken in its negative form – that is, as a prerogative of the individual to move around freely, without being hampered by others – is certainly not absolutized: under pandemic conditions, we are not free to infect others; nor are we allowed to become infected ourselves, thereby widening the circle of contagion. Each person's freedom is limited by every other person's freedom, in addition to the freedom of the community as a whole.

The value of individual life cannot be absolutized either: in extreme situations, it may be sacrificed to some cause that serves the common interest, including the defense of liberty; a life may also be voluntarily abandoned when it experiences intolerable suffering. The question raised by the pandemic, however, is not solely about individual self-determination but rather about the possibility that, under certain conditions, society may be forced to choose between saving one life and saving another – something that occurred during the pandemic's most frenetic phase. We thus enter that particularly rough territory of tragic choices that, even in peacetime, calls for the military practice of *triage*. In this situation, the conflict is not between freedom and life but between one life and another. A necessity of this sort occurred in more than one country, especially in the early months of 2020, when there were insufficient medical resources to provide life-saving treatments – especially intensive care – to a growing number of patients. Then it all became a matter of identifying a criterion for choice that responded to standards of justice, or at least equity, assuming that these kinds of words can be used in such situations.

In Northern Italy the issue of a criterion of selection was bitterly debated when the situation became particularly difficult during the first coronavirus wave: medical staff was faced with limited treatment resources, which were disproportionate with the high number of patients at risk of death. In a certain sense, a precedent did exist – that of the Taranto Steelworks – in which health was apparently opposed not to freedom but to work. In that case, in 2013, the Italian Constitutional Court proclaimed that "all the fundamental rights protected by the Constitution are mutually integrated, and it is therefore not possible to identify one of them that has primacy over the others." If this were not so, one of the rights could be expanded without limits, becoming a "tyrant" over the others. But the difference is that, as far as a highly polluting factory is concerned, it is always possible to imagine combining rights by eliminating the pollution without cutting the number of jobs; during a pandemic, however, treating one life can automatically cause the loss of another. This makes it extremely difficult to identify appropriate behavior. To avoid random choices, such as the purely chronological approach of rescuing whoever arrives first at the hospital, in spring 2020 two documents were drafted, in disagreement with each other. The first, written by the Italian Society of Anesthesiology, Analgesia, Resuscitation, and Intensive Care (SIAARTI), adopts the principle of a "greater probability of treatment success," that is, a "greater hope of life," and allows that "it could become necessary to place an age limit on admission to treatment" – effectively excluding patients who are more elderly and therefore have less hope of life.

This document was accompanied – or rather opposed – by another, drawn up by the National Committee for Bioethics, an advisory body to the Presidency of the Council of Ministers. Its view was that the clinical criterion alone is appropriate and ethically acceptable, excluding any possible discrimination based on age, gender, ethnicity, social condition, disability, or responsibility in spreading the infection. Obviously, in this case, too, choices would have to be made, but they should be based solely on the probability of the patient's recovery: "On the basis of the aforementioned indicators, the priority should be established by evaluating the parameters by which the treatment can reasonably prove to be effective, in the sense of ensuring the greatest possibility of survival." As a prerequisite to all others, the right to life cannot accept internal variations or thresholds; it is identical for everyone, regardless of any other valuation – which, in any case, can be assessed only according to clinical criteria and not by political authorities in advance of the circumstances. What policies can do – and often did not – is foresee extreme emergency situations so that we do not find ourselves on the slippery slope of "tragic choices."[11]

3

The tragic nature of the choices concerning fundamental principles – the defense of individual life and liberty – also encompasses the measures implemented during the pandemic. Despite the difference in attitude on the part of democratic and autocratic systems of government, a core question remains regarding the outcomes of the casual use of emergency declarations even in western democracies. The problem was particularly pertinent to Italy – the first country in the world to adopt a nationwide lockdown during the first and most overwhelming wave of the pandemic. Was it a "state of exception," as some maintained, or a "state of emergency," as others argued?[12] Clearly there are substantial similarities between these two states: both provide for a suspension of existing laws. But this does not mean that state of exception and state of emergency are identical. If the distinction between a "commissary dictatorship" and a "sovereign dictatorship," developed by Schmitt, is applied, then they appear to converge.[13] But it is precisely the use of Schmitt's lexicon, with its characteristic primacy of the political over the juridical, that is problematic in the case of the pandemic. Historically, especially in the first half of the last century, there were certainly more than a few crossings between the state of emergency and the state of exception (or, in Schmitt's vocabulary, between commissary dictatorship and sovereign dictatorship); and on some occasions these crossings ended up erasing the conceptual boundaries between them. When a decree-law such as an instrument of derogation from a given regulation is broadened or extended in time to the point of becoming an ordinary production of law, the state of emergency slips into that of exception and the commissary swerves toward the sovereign.

The Italian system was long vulnerable to this oscillation, because the Albertine Statute contained no reference to a state of exception or a state of emergency, but it did mention a "state of siege." To be made lawful, the state of siege had to be promulgated by the king and then approved in parliament, without any further constitutional checks. Of course, this practice, which eluded the general principle that citizen rights can be limited only through written laws, implied a primacy of the executive over the legislative that did not always end within the timeframe provided for, threatening to permanently change the balance between powers. Thus – given the far from parsimonious use of decrees issued by the prime minister during the recent pandemic in Italy – there was some fear, not unjustified, that a creeping shift might take place from a parliamentary to a governmental regime. After all, crises typically tend to centralize or verticalize decisions, concentrating all expectations on the leader. Urgency leads to shortening the timeframe for decisions, thereby investing the government with more power, proportionate to the magnitude of the perceived danger. Obviously, if the government itself assesses the severity of the danger, perhaps aided by its own appointed expert commissions, a vicious circle may result whereby the state's authority crosses the limits it has set for itself in the constitutional charter. In these kinds of situations, the government is undoubtedly tempted to strengthen its own powers and broaden the consensus it enjoys, using the crisis as an opportunity to shift the balance of power to its own advantage, away from the other constitutional bodies.

However, in distinguishing between the state of exception and the state of emergency, source and aims are more important than intensity and duration. Once the emergency has passed, the state of emergency may be a restoration of the previous system, or it may supersede it in a new constitutional regime. This alternative defines the difference between commissary and sovereign dictatorships; but, from another perspective, it also defines the difference between the state of emergency and the state of exception – which are distinct not only qualitatively but also quantitatively. The aim of the former is to rebuild a normality interrupted by unforeseen events. The latter aims to break it for the sake of a different system. Obviously, only at the end of the process does it become clear which one we are dealing with, since intermediate or partially overlapping situations are not to be excluded. There remains, however, a fundamental orientation that can be glimpsed from the beginning. This brings us to the other differentiating factor, which concerns the birth of the state of emergency or exception. In question is the relationship between constituent power and constituted power; and, even before that, the very nature of constituent power. The essential question, from which all the others follow, is whether the state is triggered by a subjective will or by an objective necessity.

Admittedly, will and necessity are not mutually exclusive and do not in principle oppose each other, since there is always a subjective evaluation that determines when the necessity arises, made by whoever is legally empowered to perform it: the head of state, the government, or the parliament. And yet it is undeniable that something evident distinguishes the realm of necessity from that of will. Whatever one may say, a catastrophic flood or an earthquake is different from a political crisis or a foreign occupation. How can one deny that a pandemic is different from a *coup d'état*, even if it cannot be ruled out that the former might provoke the latter indirectly? But if that should happen, the assessment of the exceptionality of the event would be shifted to this later stage, just as the intervention of will would relate only to it. Put simply, if it is true that the proclamation of a necessity is also the result of a decision, then there are objective parameters by which its legitimacy and appropriateness to the situation can be measured. Without losing sight of possible analogies, the decision to restore the previous order through a series of emergency measures is different from that of using an unfavorable event to overthrow it.

The person who underscored this difference in an objective emergency – which he defines as "state of siege," in line with the wording of the Albertine Statute – was Santi Romano, in a 1909 essay prompted by an earthquake in Messina and Reggio Calabria. His first concern regarding the concept of "state of siege" is to distinguish the emergency of an earthquake from that provoked by a war. Although the situation reported in Messina and Reggio Calabria was no less serious, and in some respects worse, than a military defeat, they represent essentially different cases. The urgency of intervening in the aftermath of an earthquake is hardly comparable to the police measures required in the case of popular uprisings. True, after the earthquake there were acts of looting and public disturbance that had to be suppressed. But these events are still secondary to the pressing need to "remedy the dissolution of any social and political organization caused by a completely involuntary and natural phenomenon."[14] The fact remains that a civil state of siege does not fall under a military one and therefore cannot be regulated by the war code. Instead of trying to include the earthquake state of siege in the military state of siege, the definition of "state of siege" must be extended to various situations, such as those caused by natural catastrophes. But what, asks Romano, is the basis of this extension? Is there a source of law that legitimizes the government's exceptional measures?

The answer is that it is a matter of *necessity* – which he considers a primary source of all law, as is custom; but custom is much more cogent and energetic, since it knows no limits except those established by the objective situation. Necessity is not governed by the law, as in the saying "necessity knows no law," *necessitas non habet legem*; rather it precedes and determines the law:

if it has no law, it makes it, as another common expression puts it; which means that necessity itself constitutes a genuine source of law. And it is noteworthy that its value is not restricted to the special case of government emergency powers but is much broader and has much more important and general manifestations. Necessity can be said to be the first and original source of all that is law, such that the other sources are to be considered somewhat derivative by comparison.[15]

Looking back to find the law's foundation, one must at some point stop at a first law, which draws its legitimating force solely from necessity. This remains true whether the state is instituted through a historical event or has already created its own institutions – because the necessity arises before the state, out of social needs that precede the written law. The subjective right of a state to enact the provisions that implement a state of siege arises only by reason of an objective situation. It is warranted by a mixture of necessity and contingency, not by a voluntary decision.

From this point of view, it is wrong to set the state's right to maintain its own existence against the individual freedoms of its citizens, as many do. The state of emergency – unlike the state of exception in transit toward sovereign dictatorship – does not strike against individual rights through measures that respond to catastrophic events. Admittedly, such measures may include the limitation of some freedoms – as happened during the unfortunate period we have just lived through. But, according to Romano, this limitation does not result from the state's subjective right; it comes from the regulations adopted in the act of proclaiming the state of emergency: "the state has no subjective right to exercise against that of its citizens, unless it grants it to itself through a new regulation. The relationship between the state and the citizens therefore remains mediated by this element, indeed, the relationship does not arise before this regulation is in place."[16]

4

Even if the notion of "state of exception" can be appropriately used for the measures taken in response to the pandemic, the underlying premise is certainly wrong, namely that a sovereign power was exercised with the aim of controlling and dominating our societies. I am not suggesting that no risk to democracy is lurking behind the measures taken by western governments; but this risk should be connected to a possible shift toward technocracy, and not toward the centralization of power. This is particularly important in relation to the role that politics is gradually assuming in contemporary society. What we see emerging is not a return of the political, albeit in a sovereign version, but rather a depoliticization that brings to full fruition a tendency that has long been underway. We must not confuse what, with a questionable neologism, is called "sovereignism" with an intensification of political sovereignty in a world that is instead increasingly globalized. Despite nationalistic resurgences, both the spread of the virus and the search for tools to eliminate it – especially the production of vaccines – cross widely over national borders, testifying to the need for an increasingly closer interconnection between all countries. But, at least for now, we cannot work out this interdependence through more politics: already subordinate to the dynamics of global finance, politics experienced a further setback during the pandemic when it ceded its own essential prerogative – the protection of citizens' lives – to the competence of experts. To understand this change fully, we must fit it into the two-pronged process we examined in the previous chapters: the politicization of medicine and the medicalization of politics triggered by the new immunitarian biopolitics. Once life – its preservation and development – became the main purpose of all governments, it was inevitable that upon the virus's arrival physicians would be put in charge of managing not only the health crisis but also, indirectly, every other aspect of society.

Even though the current shift is clear, this phenomenon needs to be embedded in a sequence of events that occurred over a much longer period and are linked to the relationship between politics and science as it has emerged since the beginning of the last century. An antinomic relationship soon formed between the two – at once autonomous and with mutual implications – on which Weber concentrated his research from the early 1900s on.[17] From that moment, the decline of the political became evident in the face of the economy's deterritorializing power. The sovereign paradigm performed the function of containing this power or providing it with an ideological cover for processes that, as early as after World War I, were heading in the opposite direction. Already in the first decades of the twentieth century, despite upheavals and totalitarian currents, the capitalist logic pushed politics toward a global technological–administrative order. This dynamic, by then irreversible, continued to reinforce the role of science and technology, which ultimately imposed their method onto the other languages, starting with that of politics. If politics seeks to be effective, it must, like science, realistically take into account the factual circumstances in which it is embedded. However, a difference does remain: for science to work, it must concentrate on means and exclude the realm of ends from its purview, whereas politics cannot drop them from its perspective. The technological–scientific apparatus cannot express choices regarding the type of society it anticipates, but this is precisely the objective of political action. For science to achieve its goal, it must draw a veil of ignorance not only over the future order but also over its own genesis, repressing the conditions that produced it. Conversely, politics cannot lose sight of the ends it must pursue, although it must tend to the means at its disposal with the same disenchantment as science.

Nevertheless, this distinction is soon affected by a countercurrent that breaks down the autonomy of the two spheres, placing what seems to be two separate paths back into mutual tension. On the one hand, despite its declared lack of evaluative intent, scientific research cannot be uninterested in the historical ground on which it stands – in part because of the obvious economic and political interests that it serves and depends on. On the other hand politics, occupied as it is with acquiring the resources it needs for its own action – starting with the primary resource of power – ends up concentrating on that and loses sight of its goals. At the base of both these movements, from science and from politics, lies the capitalist logic, which tends to adapt all languages to the needs of the economy. With the biopolitical turn, this picture, captured perfectly by Max Weber, suffered a further change, steered by the primacy of the preservation of life. Theorized in the early modern period by Hobbes, at a certain point this primacy became the only objective, ultimately supplanting all other values and pulling into its orbit both scientific and political interests. The epistemological shift from physics to biology that took place in the second half of the last century expresses a wider current – which I reconstructed through the genealogy of the immune paradigm. Although the immune paradigm was originally theorized in legal terms, it slid more and more in the direction of biology, and from there toward the other areas, until it became the dominant model.

There is a clear relationship between immunization and technicalization, a relationship that is becoming the dominant feature of contemporary political systems. As we have seen, it forms the backbone of what has long taken the form of an immunitarian democracy; but the pandemic has accelerated this process in a powerful way. At a time when health security had become by far the overriding concern, politics, already subordinate to economic and financial needs, was weakened even further with respect to the various interests that it should represent. In the face of a general, extraordinary problem caused by the pandemic, political conflicts gave ground to what looked like the interest of the entire citizenry: to save lives and protect the economy, which was devastated by the pandemic crisis. This was an occasion to neutralize ongoing political fights and, often, political parties themselves, which were effectively replaced by technical committees. The only legitimate interest at this point appeared to be the management of problems that affected the entire population, as opposed to the contrasting perspectives that articulate the sociopolitical dynamic. In this manner the technicians' expertise in means became so paramount as to push to the margins the discussion about ends – formerly a prerogative of politics.

The expert became the ruling figure[18] who, by virtue of his or her specialized knowledge, does not speak in the name of particular needs but on behalf of society as a whole. Although experts position themselves as mediators between science and politics, in reality their presence certifies the supremacy of the former over the latter. The government of experts, which declares itself the expression of scientific truth – even though it occupies a different place from that of bona fide scientists, who are always aware of the provisional nature of their knowledge – aims to counteract the drift toward populism, characterized by ignorance on complex questions about contemporary society. In reality, this opposition is only partly true. By shifting expertise outside parliament, which is now effectively deprived of any authority in choices that matter, this opposition creates a political deficit, in forms that ultimately acquire anti-parliamentarian, or even anti-political features. In this way, however, a technical government reduces its activity to the governance of existing resources, precluding itself from any radical action toward reform. Any government not born of political confrontation and conflict is not capable of making decisions about the future of society; it limits itself to administering it. The rupture between ends and means sanctions the silence of politics, which is neutralized by the hybrid presence of technology and economics – while only their political synthesis would allow the crisis to be tackled in an innovative way. This is why technical governments always have a conservative spirit, regardless of the parties that support them. They do indeed achieve an exit from populist regimes; but it is an exit toward the right, so to speak, because, by identifying political conflict as the risk to be avoided, they end up reproducing the populist specter of a homogeneous people. Replacing populist leaders and movements with the myth of technical expertise does not mean restoring a role to political dialectics, which represents the other exit from populism, from the left, because it puts the contest between opposing values and interests back into play.[19] Even the act of putting the pandemic behind us – in the hope that we can – hangs on this same alternative. Deluding ourselves that we can do it within the administrative confines of new economic resources will not take us very far. Only a resumption of politics, in the strongest and most powerful sense of the word, will allow us to usher in a true period of change.

5

Nothing reveals the ambivalent character of the immune system – at once protective and negative – better than Covid-19. The immune system's primary task is to protect the body from the harmful effects of the pathogenic cells that attack it: viruses, bacteria, funguses. This function is performed along two combined lines of defense. The first – expressed via innate immunity – is made up of white blood cells called phagocytes, which literally eat up the pathogenic agents, neutralizing them. The second – activated by acquired or specific immunity – is composed of specialized lymphocyte B cells, which produce antibodies; and T cells located in the thymus gland that destroy the microbial antigens by attaching to them. The immune system tackles the disease in a joint orchestration that combines, to varying degrees and with different capabilities, macrophages, lymphocytes, and neutrophils, reinstating the body's homeostatic equilibrium. The system's first manifestation is an inflammatory process – most commonly expressed as fever – which takes form in a wide variety of localized phenomena such as heat, swelling, and reddening. Although perceived as annoying symptoms to be eradicated, they actually represent the prime mode in which the immune system performs its protective function against infectious microorganisms and repairs damaged tissues. For this reason, a fever, like a helpful alarm that safeguards the body from worse damage, should be allowed to run its course rather than be immediately suppressed.

However, as the immunologist Alberto Mantovani reminds us in a book on the different types of infection,[20] inflammation can become pathological in its turn, producing cardiovascular, atherosclerotic, and even oncological diseases. Even more curious is its involvement in the infectious phenomena from which it should defend us. How can this be explained? How can the inflammatory process on the one hand protect us from infection and on the other bring it on? This apparent biological incongruity arises from the ambivalence of immune systems – of both human and social bodies – that we have explored at length. Like collective immune *dispositifs*, individual immune devices inside our body can both defend us and harm us. The problem lies in their measure, that is, in how proportional the response is to the viral attack. The moment the response goes beyond a certain threshold, established by the body's well-being, inflammation flares up, igniting a fire that is difficult to extinguish and, once it spreads to the whole body, may lead to its collapse. Everything depends on keeping the immune response under control. As long as it does not go beyond a certain limit, it performs its protective function, repairing and regenerating tissues; but, if it gets out of proportion, the damage it causes as it goes about its work is greater than the harm it is supposed to counteract; hence it amplifies this harm. Fever, for example, which is initially useful for alerting the body, beyond a certain degree destabilizes it and makes it vulnerable to the risk of implosion. What was a little flame turns into a devastating fire that risks burning down the entire organism. Similarly, the positive action of cytokines, themselves produced by the immune system, turns into a cytochemical storm[21] that threatens to overwhelm the body, causing vasodilation and circulatory shock. This is exactly what happens in Covid-19 when a blaze invades the lungs, preventing them from breathing. The damage produced by acute inflammation is not limited to bronchial obstruction – it is communicated to the kidneys, the central nervous system, the blood vessels, and the heart.[22]

At the origin of every immune excess – which is designed to reverse a necessary defense into a devastating autoimmune disease – there is a sort of "mistake" or, we might say, an "oversight" – not because the immune system sees too little, but because it sees too much. Instead of staying blind to its internal components, it recognizes them and, directing its aim at them, turns its fire against itself. This oversight – this failure to distinguish between self and not-self, or between self and other – has been the focus of immunological research for decades and a seemingly inexplicable enigma from the start. *Horror autotoxicus* is how Paul Ehrlich defined it in the early twentieth century,[23] using a term indicative of how difficult it is for us to accept a self-toxic mechanism, a process that produces antibodies directed against the same organism. The notion that resisted conceptualization was that of an auto-antibody: something that neutralizes antibodies instead of blocking antigens. This recursive effect is generated whenever the immune system, failing to overlook its own components, identifies and targets them. Rather than turning outward, the immune system attacks the very cells it generated, empowering the infection it is meant to extinguish. Thus, we ourselves – our organic elements – become the target of our own defenses.

Half a century was to pass before immunology got to the bottom of this literally antinomic self-aggression, when autoimmune diseases began to be studied in the 1940s. These kinds of illnesses are not pathologies refractory to the immune system's action, as was once thought, but one of its perverse effects; hence the use of drugs, called immunosuppressants, which began to be used to block or reduce an excessive and thus harmful immune response. But – confirming the complexity of the immune *dispositif* – the first defenses against this superabundance of immunization are induced by the immune system itself, which self-corrects, so to speak, when it realizes that it is out of control. For example, anti-inflammatory cytokines have the role of "firefighters" against the very blazes that they started. Similarly, in response to an excessive reaction, the regulatory T cells act as inhibitory brakes against undue acceleration, while a kind of biological extinguisher cools down the inflammation. The thymus plays a particularly important role in this extremely complicated process, by eliminating parts of the autoreactive cells and clearing the field of their debris.

Of course, the immune system's self-control – the containment it exercises over its own aggressive power – is limited and imperfect. Something always escapes the surveillance organs, risking a new systemic crisis. As the experience of Covid-19 has taught us, success in treating the disease in some patients does not mean that we have learned to cure it in other, dramatically more serious cases. This is partly due to the fact that, while the immune system requires immunosuppressants to reduce its own excesses, it cannot be weakened to the point of remaining defenseless against the virus. This makes it particularly difficult to cure autoimmune diseases. Today, immunosuppressant drugs, while still used, are accompanied and in part replaced by biologic drugs such as monoclonal antibodies, which present fewer risks. In any case, the aim of reducing the production of antibodies is to re-establish the homeostatic equilibrium by remodulating the immune reaction.

The truth is that, as has been argued,[24] a condition of perfect equilibrium is never attainable, since the immune cells and molecules are constantly moving around to repair any damage produced, and this leads to further transformation within our tissues. Accordingly, the temporary loss of an initial equilibrium becomes the condition for being able to renew it again and again over time. At stake in this chain of actions and reactions is not just the relationship with external microbes, as portrayed in a reductive conception of the immune system, but also the relationship with the internal microbial colony. One of the functions of the immune system is a cognitive capacity to make information circulate among even distant elements, putting them in relation with one another. Of course, its essential function, more necessary today than ever before, remains the production of molecules designed to block the circulation of viruses. But we would be wrong to see it as a simple defensive barrier, when its most complex task lies in a sort of continuous negotiation with the organism's internal and external worlds. In an activity that never pauses, a functioning immune system unites maximum sensitivity with precision of the highest kind: sensitivity in detecting the presence of even minimal but potentially harmful pathogenic elements, and precision in the capacity to distinguish them from other microorganisms that are useful to the organism. Speaking of this, we must not forget the extraordinary fact that human beings themselves are largely made up of microbes, whose elimination would have very serious consequences for the organic system. The microbial colony residing in the intestine, for example, plays a necessary role in mediating between the gastrointestinal tract and the central nervous system. In short, contrary to the paradigmatic opposition between community and immunity, the immune system, examined in its various ambient components, can be likened to a community formed by many different individuals, each of which has a different role, indispensable to the life of the whole.[25]

6

We all know that war is used repeatedly as a metaphor in descriptions of the pandemic. Enemy, heroism, trenches, weapons, munitions, defenses – these words have been used hand over fist during the past two years, by politicians and journalists but also by physicians and healthcare workers, to describe the ongoing fight with the virus. Against this indiscriminate use and regardless of whether the comparison is apt, some have pointed out that the language of war is in itself divisive. It might be opportune to appeal instead to unity and civil solidarity in the face of adversity. There has also been some concern that this "state of siege" jargon might make us less responsive to the creeping authoritarianism of the government's pandemic-containing measures.[26] To what extent these observations hit the mark, or whether they too are the result of excessive scaremongering about common language, remains debatable. What has in any case gone unmentioned is that this military lexicon is inherent in the immune paradigm. The use of war images in medicine is well known; but what must be stressed is the singular importance of this use for immunological science. As mentioned, nothing better than military terminology has been found, over decades now, to describe the immune system's protective role against pathogenic agents. The immunization process has been translated into the language of a real war, in which the survival of the body is at stake; and the fight is carried out by the army of antibodies against the invading microorganisms.

We know the historical and epistemological context of this semantic transmigration from the legal–political to the medical–biological side of the immune paradigm: the fight against major infectious diseases and the prevailing socio-Darwinian ideology. But there is also the context, which we could characterize as philosophical, of a conception of biological immunity built around the opposition between self and not-self. This was theorized for the first time by the great immunologist Frank Macfarlane Burnet: "Antibody production or any other type of immunological reaction is against foreign material – against something that is not self."[27] Subsequent events, such as the eruption of AIDS, reinforced this polemological interpretation of the immune system, at once defensive and offensive, which was destined to intersect ever more emphatically with the contemporary biopolitical lexicon. More than an evolutionary process or a systemic picture of relationships, what lies at its core is the biological identity of the individual organism, understood as a monad, to be preserved unchanged against external attacks, by being isolated from the surrounding environment. Conceived of by analogy with the psychic identity, it acquires an almost metaphysical configuration – a corporeal unit corresponding fully to the spiritual nucleus of the person who inhabits it.

From the very beginning, however, this conception clashed with a problem difficult to solve, which is about the contours of the immune system itself. Once the antibodies are activated by antigens, it was asked, how do they not impact the inner components of the organism as well? The only way to explain the puzzle from within these assumptions was to imagine that the immune system did not "see" or "tolerate" them, but limited itself to attacking the pathogens that came from outside. Since it remained blind or mute toward its own body, this meant that it was defined in essentially negative terms – like something that works only as long as it refrains from fully exercising its role. This passive idea of immunity fails to answer a two-pronged question about allogenic transplants, long considered impossible, and autoimmune diseases, which are difficult to understand within this interpretive framework.

The only way to arrive at an answer was to shift the focus of immunological science from the preservation of individual integrity to the evolution of identity, following the perspective opened by Mechnikov, who, as we saw, arrived at the Pasteur Institute in the late 1800s. Thinking about the immunization process as dynamic rather than restorative, he viewed the immune *dispositif* not as a barrier against the external environment but as a filter through which one could interact with it. From this perspective – described of course in terms that were still immature, and for this reason long marginalized in immunology studies in its day – the individual body appeared not as a closed entity but as a construct that evolved over time, subject to continuous transformations within a "social community" – or, as Burnet evocatively called it, a climax community. This would make it possible a few decades later to understand tolerance – necessary for organ transplants, but also for keeping the fetus safe inside the mother's womb – not as a blind spot in the immune system but as an active learning capacity developed during the embryonic stage. According to the theory of clonal selection, the elimination of self-reactive clones is what protects the body from self-disintegration. Furthermore, this shifting of the concept of immunity from a negative to a positive meaning made it possible for allogenic transplants to be not resisted by the immune system but rather supported under certain conditions. As Peter Medawar argued, if the organism is trained, it can even learn to recognize some foreign components as its own, which allows for transplants without the use of immunosuppressants, since it is the immune system itself that mediates this operation.[28] This means that tolerance should not be thought of as a non-immunity – an immune deficiency – but rather as a sort of reverse immunity, which works for and against itself at the same time.

This new research, destined to offer an image of immunity radically different from the purely defensive one, intersected in the 1970s with Niels Jerne's network theory, most notably in the autonomous network theory version coming out of the Paris school. According to a cognitive type of interpretation that highlights the immune system's self-reflective character, this system would appear also to contain apparently external elements. Thus, with the passing of the traditional opposition between self and non-self or proper and improper, antigen and antibody – now defined respectively as "epitopes" and "paratopes" – can exchange roles: "the immune system is an enormous and complex network of paratopes that recognize sets of idiotopes, and of idiotopes that are recognized by sets of paratopes."[29] Despite the risk of a mentalistic drift that would lead the entire reality back to the reflective field of the self, the self does end up being constitutively altered, and thus indistinguishable from the alterity that it carries within itself and with which it interacts continuously. Once the preliminary condition was dropped – the assumption that the system must not recognize itself lest it destroy itself – researchers were able to turn it upside down, into the idea that the immune system does nothing but recognize itself, but starting from a visual angle that no longer distinguishes between self and other. As Alfred Tauber concludes, in a book that admirably retraces this complex and fascinating story, "the immune system must not only function to identify itself as opposed to the other, but also constantly define self from itself. On such a basis immunity is a *process* that always provides for an open system of self-definition, constantly producing self and other from itself."[30]

This was a profound change in the biological immune paradigm, a change that has been reinforced over recent decades. Far from being a discriminatory barrier against the external environment, the immune system is now seen as that which, under certain conditions, facilitates a relationship with the outside. A static, exclusionary model has given way to one that is dynamic and inclusive – in some respects, more communitarian than immunitarian. The self is not something that precedes immunization, calling upon it for defense, but rather its outcome, a product of the fruitful intersection of identity and otherness – an identity that is othered from the outset.[31] Two ideas from Burnet's model come tumbling down: one, that the organism does not produce immune responses against its own components; and two, that it produces responses against every external component. Autoimmunity – which must be distinguished from self-reactivity and, even more so, from autoimmune illnesses – is not a pathology but a biological *dispositif* present in all living beings, and one that plays a crucial role even in their homeostasis. All organisms contain foreign elements inside themselves – examples are fetuses in mothers, but also bacteria and microorganisms;

and these elements actually make up a large part of them. Illness does not arise when an external element enters inside an organism – this is the norm, not the exception – but when it negatively affects the organism's homeostatic development. Ninety percent of the living being is made up of bacteria; only ten percent consists of cells that carry its genome. For this reason, it could well be said that each one of us is ten times more "other" than self.[32] It is true that some bacteria are harmful, but not all of them are. Most of them are indifferent or useful to human beings – just as human beings are useful to them, for that matter. Rather than an individual, a human being is an ecosystem composed of different, integrated species – a sort of common immunity or co-immunity,[33] formed by a colony of symbionts that have an indispensable function in the metabolism, in repairing and regenerating tissues. Without indulging in the idea that biodiversity, by itself, protects against disease, we must also guard against imagining that it produces disease.

7

The inextricable relationship between immunity and community is not hidden solely in the folds of our immune system. It is also inscribed in the relationships that bind or divide human beings affected by a pandemic. What appeared to be a paradigmatic opposition – between *communitas* and *immunitas* – was suddenly revealed during the pandemic to be what it has always been, that is, a dialectic in which one term is indistinguishable from the other. From time immemorial, as we have seen, neither acquires meaning outside their relationship. Historically, there has never been a non-immunized community, just as immunization is a *dispositif* common to all individuals and all societies. Nevertheless, this does not detract from an essential distinction that has profoundly marked our history. While community unites its members by putting them in the same condition, immunity divides its members into those who possess it and those who do not. We have seen how this division cuts across all spheres, from the legal to the social, from the technological to the biomedical. This is where the logical and etymological opposition with community comes back into view. While community, understood in its universalistic sense, evokes equality, immunity takes the form of a privilege: those who are immune, by virtue of their special status, are freed from the bond, or risk, of a common situation.

The pandemic threw this centuries-old arrangement – the relationship between immunity and privilege – into radical crisis. Spreading rapidly throughout the world, the virus unified it in a condition that seemed impossible to escape on the basis of distinctions of ethnicity, gender, social level, or power.[34] In a certain sense, it recreated the original *communitas*, defined by exposure to otherness and to the contact that this brings with it. Of course, under the pressure of an ill, this status presents itself in the extremely negative terms we have all experienced. But, through the nets of pain and suffering, it allows glimpses into a vulnerability that harkens back to the constitutive characteristics of the human species. With a violence no one was prepared for, the immune threshold set by modern civilization itself was suddenly lowered, or it even collapsed. The immune system of individual bodies and that of social bodies, which had constituted for centuries a solid protective barrier, appeared incapable of reacting effectively against the virus's attacks. The only possible response to defend a community exposed to the virus was to trigger an artificial immunization, however primitive, by separating individuals into rigidly confined spaces. The expression "social distancing" – used without full awareness of the semantic paradox it implies – tells us something about what it means to defend a community by dismembering it. Social distancing reinforces a mode of action implicit in the processes of modernization, which unifies society in the form of the separation of its individuals: it divides human beings in order to save a society threatened by the virus.

This first defensive stage, expressed as individual confinement, is acceptable only within certain limits and, most importantly, for a given period – not otherwise. It was followed by a second, much more effective immune *dispositif*, which consisted of the vaccine. In this case, too, immunity and community crossed paths in an unprecedented way. The vaccine, the most classic instrument of immunization, became the most necessary common good. For the first time in the history of the world, the entire planet, not just one part of the community, demanded immunization. The prospect of immunizing the whole world had never even been imagined before then. The full significance of this historic turning point is difficult to fathom. We are in a transition that – it bears repeating – is making community and immunity coincide for the first time in history, changing immunity from a blade that cuts through community into its selfsame form. This turning point, inconceivable until now, was made possible not by an ethical choice – although some were made, here and there – but by a convergence of interests that makes clear that this time, for the first time, one part of the world cannot be saved without saving all of it at the same time. Certainly the environmental crisis has produced a similar impression in the past few decades. In this case, too, the ecological transition that it demands and makes inevitable will either be global or not happen at all. But it moves with less intensity and at a slower pace than the pandemic. While the risk related to the environmental crisis still appears to most people as a possibility, questioned by some but in any case postponed, the risk related to the coronavirus has impressed itself onto the consciousness of billions of people as risk of an atrocious death or, at best, of an illness with unpredictable and certainly harmful consequences.

Accordingly, the demand for a common immunity has come not only from peoples but also from state governments, because these are aware of the danger implicit in excluding even a single country from vaccination. The only possibility we have of withstanding the disease is if the world arrives, as one, at "herd immunity" – which is also referred to as "common immunity." However, this need for general immunity, although expressed emphatically by heads of state at international summits, has hardly received an adequate response in the real world. According to the World Health Organization, herd immunity cannot be reached in 2021 for the following reasons, listed in *Nature*:[35] vaccination is not proceeding uniformly in all countries; the spread of variants could upend it; we do not know how long vaccine immunity lasts; vaccinated people's return to risky behaviors could give new life to the pandemic.

The dialectics – the confluence and clash – between community and immunity is not destined to arrive at a definitive resolution. The negative, held back and at the same time produced by immune *dispositifs*, does not disappear completely but re-emerges in ever new forms. The world was unified first by the overwhelming spread of the virus and later by the demand for immunity that it generated; but, once the vaccine was produced, the global community was immediately furrowed by new lines of separation caused by very different chances of gaining access to it – both within individual countries, which are divided by vaccination timings and methods, and among countries, which are in turn separated into haves and have-nots. Unbridgeable differences, mended by the emergency, split open again between the First, the Second, and the Third World. Even among the wealthiest and most technologically advanced regions, which received the initial and most widespread distribution of the vaccine, there remained a difference between self-producing countries and countries that had to wait to purchase the vaccine according to their means. The gap between the overall need for billions of doses and the available supplies is astounding. Even bigger is the gap between the stocks held by the richest countries, which reaches almost 90 percent, and the incredibly slim amount held by the poorest. It is estimated that the African continent has received a minimal portion of the vaccines produced. From this point of view, the instrument that was potentially designed to reduce inequalities through global immunization now risks multiplying them, reproducing immunization's initially divisive and exclusionary character. Far from coinciding with *communitas*, *immunitas* is detaching itself from it again, regressing toward its original meaning of privilege.[36] What divides the different regions of the world is not only their economic but also their technological capacities – the lack of adequate know-how that still affects the vast majority of countries, as opposed to the few that have monopolized vaccine production and left the others with the alternative of either falling deeper into poverty in order to purchase vaccines or surrendering to the virus.

At the heart of the matter lies not only the relationship between countries but also that between governments and the giants of the pharmaceutical industry – an industry known to act in defense of its profits, as was predictable. A clash has broken out over patent waivers and the granting of licenses, and an extensive number of public and private stakeholders have joined the fray. Since the pharmaceutical industry is in good part interlaced with government agencies, this standoff cannot be reduced to a disagreement between governments and big pharma. Good intentions will certainly not be enough to resolve it, seeing that interests continue to diverge. Drug producers have put forward several reasons, backed by some governments, for rejecting the proposed measures: on the one hand, waiving intellectual property rights disincentivizes private financing; on the other, poor countries have insufficient technological equipment to cope with an increase in large-scale production. But in the face of the magnitude and novelty of the global pandemic, both justifications appear specious and inadequate. Obviously, pharmaceutical industry share prices cannot be allowed to crash in the stock market, and the export blockade that the United States and the United Kingdom, above all, have set up on their own production must be removed. But this does not diminish the fact that the cost of vaccines for weaker buyers can and should be drastically lowered. As always with conflicts that cannot be resolved through negotiation, the issue is not just economic or technological in nature but political. Never more than in this case must politics impose itself over all other motives. If the logic of profit prevails, the game will be lost before it has even been played. If, instead, politics is revitalized by an otherwise ungovernable situation and is able to assert itself, the battle, however difficult, can at least be fought. Never more than today, in the throes of a biopolitical regime, has politics been concerned with the protection and development of life – not just of individual populations but of the human species as a whole. When community and immunity rediscover a shared boundary, the life of each is protected only by the life of all.

Notes

Notes to Introduction

1 Visit https://gbdeclaration.org.
2 Visit https://www.johnsnowmemo.com/john-snow-memo.html.
3 Roberto Esposito, *Immunitas: The Protection and Negation of Life*, trans. by Z. Hanafi. Cambridge: Polity, 2011.

Notes to Chapter 1

1 See R. Esposito, *Communitas: The Origin and Destiny of Community*, trans. by T. Campbell. Stanford, CA: Stanford University Press, 2009. The etymology of *munus* and its derivatives is discussed in the introduction.
2 R. Esposito, *Immunitas: The Protection and Negation of Life*, trans. by Z. Hanafi. Cambridge: Polity, 2011. For a recent examination of the immune paradigm, see S. Spina, *Immunitas e persona*. Pisa: ETS, 2020.
3 See F. Tönnies, *Community and Society*, trans. by C. P. Loomis. London: Routledge, 2017
4 Regarding the dialectics between politics and biology within the immune paradigm, see I. Mutsaers, *Immunological Discourse in Political Philosophy: Immunisation and Its Discontents*. London: Routledge, 2016.

5 On the genealogy of the immune paradigm, see the broad-ranging, careful study by E. Cohen, *A Body Worth Defending: Immunity, Biopolitics and the Apotheosis of the Modern Body*. Duhram, NC: Duke University Press, 2009.

6 Regarding the use of war metaphors to describe the immune system, see P. Jaret, "Our immune system: The wars within," *National Geographic*, 169 (1986): 702–35.

7 Regarding the transformative power of political metaphors in defining biological immunity, see E. S. Golub, "Semiosis for the immune system but not the immune response, or what can be learned about language by studying the immune system?" in *The Semiotics of Cellular Communication in the Immune System*, ed. by E. E. Sercarz, F. Celada, N. A. Mitchison and T. Tada. Berlin: Springer, 1988, pp. 65–9; F. Karush, "Metaphors in Immunology," in *Immunology, 1930–1980: Essays on the History of Immunology*, ed. by P. Mazumdar. Toronto: Wall & Thompson, 1989, pp. 73–80; and especially E. Martin, *Flexible Bodies: The Role of Immunity in American Culture, from the Days of Polio to the Age of AIDS*. Boston, MA: Beacon Press, 1994.

8 For a history of legal immunity, see especially L. S. Frey and M. L. Frey, *The History of Diplomatic Immunity*. Columbus: Ohio State University Press, 1999; G. McClanahan, *Diplomatic Immunity: Principles, Practices, Problem*. London: C. Hurt, 1989.

9 See Cohen, *A Body Worth Defending*, pp. 41ff.

10 See M. Harrison, *Disease and the Modern World: From 1500 to the Present Day*. Cambridge: Polity, 2004; J. N. Hays, *The Burden of Disease: Epidemics and Human Response in Western History*. New Brunswick, NJ: Rutgers University Press, 2009 [1988]; S. Morand, *La prochaine peste: Une histoire globale des maladies infectieuses*. Paris: Fayard, 2016; M. D. Grmek, *Pathological Realities: Essays on Disease, Experiments and History*, edited by P.-O. Méthot. New York: Fordham University Press, 2019.

11 J. Diamond, *Guns, Germs, and Steel: The Fates of Human Societies*. New York: W. W. Norton, 1997, p. 77.

12 On this topic, see N. Gualde, *Les microbes aussi ont une histoire: Des épidémies de peste aux menaces de guerre bactériologique*. Paris: Empêcheurs de penser en ronde, 2003, especially pp. 203ff. On the decimation of the American peoples caused by epidemics, see H. Dobyns, *Their Number Become Thinned*. Knoxwille: University of Toronto Press, 1983; J. W. Verano and D. H. Ubelaker, eds., *Disease and Demography in the*

Americas. Washington, DC: Smithsonian Institution, 1992; A. F. Ramenofsky, *Vectors of Death: Archaeology of European Contact*. Albuquerque: University of New Mexico Press, 1987; R. Thornton, *American Indian Holocaust and Survival: A Population History since 1492*, Norman, OK: University of Oklahoma Press, 1987; A. Crosby, *The Columbian Exchange: Biological and Cultural Consequences of 1942*, Westport, CT: Praeger, 2003.

13 On the Spanish conquest of the Aztec Empire, see H. Thomas, *Conquest: Montezuma, Cortés and the Fall of Old Mexico*. New York: Simon & Schuster, 1993; B. Levy, *Conquistador: Hernán Cortés, King Montezuma, and the Last Stand of Aztecs*. New York: Bantam Books, 2008; C. Todorov, *La conquête de l'Amérique: La question de l'autre*. Paris: Seuil, 2013.

14 See J. Ruffié, *De la biologie à la culture*. Paris: Flammarion, 1976; J. Ruffié and J.-C. Sournia, *Les épidémies dans l'histoire de l'homme: De la peste au SIDA*. Paris: Flammarion, 1976.

15 M. Foucault, *The Birth of the Clinic: An Archaeology of Medical Perception*, trans. by A. M. Sheridan. London: Routledge, 2003, p. 24.

16 Foucault, *Birth of the Clinic*, p. 33.

17 M. Foucault, "The birth of social medicine" [1974], trans. by R. Hurley, in *Essential Works of Foucault 1954–1984*, vol. 3: *Power*, ed. by J. Faubion. New York: New Press, 2000, 134–56, here p. 137.

18 M. Foucault, "The crisis of medicine or the crisis of anti-medicine?" trans. by E. C. Knowlton, Jr., W. J. King, and C. O'Farrell. *Foucault Studies*, 1 (2004): 5–19, here p. 14. DOI: https://doi.org/10.22439/fs.v0i1.562.

19 M. Foucault, "The birth of social medicine" [1974], trans. by R. Hurley, in *Essential Works of Foucault 1954–1984*, vol. 3: *Power*, ed. by J. Faubion. New York: New Press, 2000, p. 144.

20 Foucault, "Birth of social medicine," p. 153.

21 For a history of vaccination, see J.-F. de Raymond, *La querelle de l'inoculation ou préhistoire de la vaccination*. Paris: Vrin, 1982; H. Bazin, *Vaccination: A History from Lady Montagu to Jenner and Genetic Engineering*. Montrogue: John Libbey Eurotext, 2011; S. Plotkin, ed., *History of Vaccine Development*. New York: Springer, 2011.

22 C. Mather, *The Angel of Bethesda*, ed. by G. W. Jones. Barre, MA: American Antiquarian Society and Barre Publishers, 1972 [1724].

23 E. Jenner, *An Inquiry into the Causes and Effects of the variolae vaccinae: A Disease Discovered in Some of the Western*

Counties of England, Particularly Gloucestershire, and Known by the Name of Cow Pox. London: S. Cooley Gosnell, 1808 [1798].

24 Foucault, "Birth of social medicine," p. 155.

25 Foucault, "Birth of social medicine," p. 155, translation modified.

26 See N. Brown, *Immunitary Life: A Biopolitics of Immunity.* London: Palgrave Macmillan, 2019, esp. the chapter "Spherologies of immunisation," pp. 169–214. On the politics of vaccination and the conflicts it has given rise to, see D. Brunton, *The Politics of Vaccination: Practice and Policy in England, Wales, Ireland, Scotland.* Rochester, NY: University of Rochester, 2008; S. Blume, "Anti-vaccination movements and their interpretations," *Social Science and Medicine*, 62 (2006): 628–42; J. Colgrove, "The ethics and politics of compulsory HPV vaccination," *New England Journal of Medicine*, 355 (2006): 2389–91; N. Durbach, *Bodily Matters: The Anti-Vaccination Movement in England, 1853–1907.* Durham, NC: Duke University Press, 2004; B. L. Hausman, "Immunity, modernity, and biopolitics of vaccination resistence," *Configurations*, 25 (2017): 279–300.

27 See C. Richet, *Discours: Centenaire de Louis Pasteur: L'Institut Pasteur de Lille et la célébration du centenaire de Pasteur à Lille.* Lille: G. Marquart, 1922. On Pasteur in general, see A. Cadeddu, *Dal mito alla storia: Biologia e medicina in Pasteur.* Milan: Angeli, 1991.

28 B. Latour, *The Pasteurization of France*, trans. by A. Sheridan and J. Law. Cambridge, MA: Harvard University Press, 1988, p. 40. See also B. Latour and S. Woolgar, *La vie de laboratoire.* Paris: La Découverte, 1988; and M. Morange, ed., *L'Institut Pasteur: Contribution à son histoire.* Paris: La Découverte, 1991.

29 Latour, *The Pasteurization of France*, p. 48.

30 Latour, *The Pasteurization of France*, p. 58.

31 On the clash between Pasteur and Koch, see K. C. Carter, "The Koch–Pasteur dispute on establishing the cause of anthrax," *Bulletin of the History of Medicine*, 62 (1988): 42–57; M. Crosland, "Science and the Franco-Prussian War," *Social Studies of Science*, 6 (1976): 185–214.

32 For the French edition, see F.-A. Pouchet, *Hétérogénie, ou Traité de la génération spontanée, basé sur de nouvelles expériences.* Paris: Baillière et fils, 1859. On the controversy about spontaneous generation, seee J. Farley, *The Spontaneous Generation Controversy from Descartes to Oparin.* Baltimore, MD: Johns

Hopkins University Press, 1974; N. Roll-Hansen, 'Experimental method and spontaneous generation: The controversy between Pasteur and Pouchet, 1859–64, *Journal of the History of Medicine*, 34 (1979): 273–92; J. Farley and G. Geison, "Le débat entre Pasteur et Pouchet: Science, politique et génération spontanée, au xixème siècle en France," in *La science telle qu'elle se fait*, ed. by M. Callon and B. Latour. Paris: La Découverte, 991, pp. 87–145.

33 A. Silverstein, "Cellular versus Humoral Immunity: Determinants and Consequences of an Epic Nineteenth-Century Battle," in his *A History of Immunology*. San Diego, CA: Academic Press, 1989, 38–58. More generally on the conflicts between the "microbe hunters," see the book by P. de Kruif, *Microbe Hunters*. San Diego, CA: Harcourt Brace Jovanovich, 1926, which is still useful.

34 A.-M. Moulin, *Le dernier langage de la medicine: Histoire de l'immunologie de Pasteur au Sida*. Paris: PUF, 1991, p. 69 (translated here from the original).

35 See É. Metchnikoff, *Immunity in Infective Diseases*. Cambridge: Cambridge University Press, 1905. On the extraordinary importance of Mechnikov's research, see A. I. Tauber, *The Immune Self: Theory or Metaphor?* Cambridge: Cambridge University Press, 1997.

36 See Ilya Ilyich Mechnikov, Nobel Lecture, December 11, 1908, in *Nobel Lectures in Physiology or Medicine 1901–1921*. Amsterdam: Elsevier Publishing Company, 1967, pp. 281–300.

Notes to Chapter 2

1 A. Brossat, *La démocratie immunitaire*. Paris: La Dispute, 2003, p. 10; the remark by Ernest Renan can be found in *Recollections of My Youth*, trans. by C. B. Pitman. London: Chapman and Hall Ltd., 1883, p. xx (Preface).

2 B. Constant, "The liberty of ancients compared with that of moderns," trans. by B. Fontana, in B. Constant, *Political Writings*. Cambridge: Cambridge University Press, 1988, 307–8, here p. 310; translation modified.

3 Brossat, La démocratie immunitaire, p. 16.

4 See E. Canetti, *Crowds and Power*, trans. by C. Stewart. New York: Seabury, 1960 and pp. 17–19 in the Italian translation: *Massa e potere*. Milan: Adelphi, 1981.

5 On this topic, see A. D. Napier, *The Age of Immunology:*

Conceiving a Future in an Alienating World. Chicago, IL: University of Chicago Press, 2003.

6 Jacques Derrida, *Rogues: Two Essays on Reason*, trans. by Pascale-Anne Brault and Michael Naas. Stanford, CA: Stanford University Press, 2005, p. 37.

7 Derrida, *Rogues*, p. 52.

8 Derrida, *Rogues*, p. 53.

9 See especially the second, definitive article in Immanuel Kant, *Perpetual Peace: A Philosophical Essay* [1795], trans. with introduction and notes by M. Campbell Smith, London: George Allen & Unwin, 1903

10 Derrida, *Rogues*, p. 33.

11 Derrida, *Rogues*, p. 35.

12 Derrida, *Rogues*, p. 37.

13 Derrida, *Rogues*, p. 72.

14 On this topic, see A. Schiavone, *Non ti delego: Perché abbiamo smesso di credere nella loro politica*. Milan: Rizzoli, 2013, pp. 31ff.

15 See G. Carillo, "Nel molto c'è il tutto: La democrazia nel dibattito sui regimi politici (Erodoto, III, 80, 1–6)," in *Oltre la democrazia: Un itinerario attraverso i classici*, ed. by G. Duso, Rome: Carocci, 2004, pp. 31–53.

16 L. Canfora, *Democracy in Europe: A History of an Ideology*, trans. by S. Jones. Oxford: Blackwell, 2006, pp. 7–8.

17 Canfora, *Democracy in Europe*, p. 5.

18 Canfora, *Democracy in Europe*, p. 5.

19 A. Gramsci, *Selections from Prison Notebooks: The Modern Prince*, ed. and trans. by Q. Hoare and G. N. Smith. London: ElecBook, 1999, p. 423; translation modified.

20 L. Canfora, *Critica della retorica democratica*. Rome-Bari: Laterza, 2002, p. 63.

21 Canfora, *Critica della retorica democratica*, p. 66.

22 G. Duso has argued particularly persuasively about these antinomies in the modern concept of democracy; see his "Genesi e aporie dei concetti della democrazia moderna," in *Oltre la democrazia: Un itinerario attraverso i classici*, ed. by G. Duso, Rome: Carocci, 2004, pp. 107–38. But see also *Filosofia politica*, 3 (2006), an issue dedicated to the headword *democrazia*.

23 B. Manin, *The Principles of Representative Government*. New York: Cambridge University Press, 1997. See on this subject B. Karsenti, *Elezione e giudizio di tutti*, in *Filosofia politica*, 3 (2006): 415–30.

24 J.-J. Rousseau, *The Social Contract* [1762], 4.3.2. [See Montesquieu, *The Spirit of Laws*, 2.2.]

25 See E.-J. Sieyès, *Dire de l'Abbé Sieyès sur la question du veto royal (7-9-1789)*. Versailles: Baudoin Imprimeur de l'Assemblée Nationale, 1789.

26 J.-J. Rousseau, *The Government of Poland* [1783], trans. with introduction and notes by Willmoore Kendall, preface by Harvey C. Mansfield, Jr. Indianapolis, IN: Hackett Publishing Company, 1985.

27 B. Manin, *The Principles of Representative Government*. New York: Cambridge University Press, 1997, p. 182.

28 Manin, *Principles of Representative Government*, p. 142.

29 C. Schmitt, *Constitutional Theory*, ed. and trans. by Jeffrey Seitzer. Durham, NC: Duke University Press, 2007, p. 284.

30 Rousseau, Social Contract 3.15.5 (*elle [la souveranité] consiste essentiellement dans la volonté générale, et la volonté ne se réprésente point: elle est la même, ou elle est autre; il n'y a point de milieu*).

31 Rousseau, *Social Contract*, 1.6.7.

32 Rousseau, *Social Contract*, 1.6.9.

33 J.-J. Rousseau, *Émile or Treatise on Education*, translated by B. Foxley. London: J. M. Dent, 1911, p. 7 (book i).

34 Rousseau, *Social Contract*, 2.7.3.

35 Rousseau, *Social Contract*, 3.4.1.

36 H. Arendt, *On Revolution*. London: Penguin, 1990, p. 77.

37 Arendt, *On Revolution*, p. 78.

38 Arendt, *On Revolution*, p. 79.

39 Arendt, *On Revolution*, p. 97.

40 C. Schmitt, *Volksentscheid und Volksbegehren: Ein Beitrag zur Auslegung der Weimarer Verfassung und zur Lehre von der unmittelbaren Demokratie*. Berlin: De Gruyter, 1927, pp. 33–4, as translated in G. Agamben, *The Kingdom and the Glory: For a Theological Genealogy of Economy and Government*, trans. by L. Chiesa with M. Mandarini. Stanford, CA: Stanford University Press, 2011, p. 171.

41 Schmitt, *Volksentscheid und Volksbegehren*, p. 34, as translated in Agamben, *The Kingdom and the Glory*, p. 172.

42 Carl Schmitt, *The Crisis of Parliamentary Democracy*, trans. by E. Kennedy. Cambridge, MA: MIT Press, 1988, p. 28.

43 On this topic, see B. de Giovanni, *Alle origini della democrazia di massa: I filosofi e i giuristi*. Naples: Editoriale Scientifica, 2013.

44 C. Schmitt, *Constitutional Theory*, ed. and trans. by Jeffrey Seitzer. Durham, NC: Duke University Press, 2007, p. 270.

45 Schmitt, *Constitutional Theory*, p. 276.
46 See R. Esposito, "Democrazia" [1993], in his *Dieci pensieri sulla politica*. Bologna: il Mulino, 2011, pp. 55–78.
47 On the necessity for this equilibrium, see N. Urbinati, "La democrazia rappresentativa e i suoi critici," in *Democrazia: Storia e teoria di un'esperienza filosofica e politica*, ed. by C. Altini. Bologna: il Mulino, 2011, pp. 219–54.
48 A. de Tocqueville, *Democracy in America*, ed. and trans. by H. C. Mansfeld and D. Winthorp. Chicago, IL: University of Chicago Press, 2000, 2.2.5 (= Book 2, Section 2, Chapter 5, "Of the Use That Americans Make of Association in Civil Life"; p. 492).
49 Tocqueville, *Democracy in America*, 2.2.5 (p. 489).
50 Arendt, *On Revolution*, p. 153.
51 Arendt, *On Revolution*, p. 168.
52 Arendt, *On Revolution*, p. 156.
53 Arendt, *On Revolution*, pp. 267–8.
54 É. Balibar, "Democracy after its decline: Some hypotheses." Paper presented at the conference *Rewiring Democracy: Beyond "Us" and "Them,"* La Maison Française & Nuyorican Poets Café, NYU, November 8, 2019.

Notes to Chapter 3

1 Regarding the growing importance of the notion of "biopolitics," see especially T. Campbell and A. Sitze, eds., *Biopolitics: A Reader*. Durham, NC: Duke University Press, 2013; P. Ticineto Clough and C. Willse, eds., *Beyond Biopolitics: Essays on the Governance of Life and Death*. Durham, NC: Duke University Press, 2011; M. Vatter, *The Republic of Living: Biopolitics and the Critique of Civil Society*. New York: Fordham, 2014; S. E. Wilmer and A. Zukauskaite, eds., *Resisting Biopolitics: Philosophical, Political and Performative Strategies*. New York: Routledge, 2016; L. Bazzicalupo, *Biopolitica: Una mappa concettuale*, Rome: Carocci, 2010; Y.-C. Zarka, 'Biopolitique du coronavirus', *Citées*, 84 (2020): n.p.
2 J.-L. Nancy, "La sindrome biopolitica," *MicroMega* 8 (2020): 56–61, here p. 57.
3 F. Warin, "La flamme d'une chandelle: La biopolitique en question," which can be found on the author's site, at bit.ly/3eG B5gL; alternatively, visit http://allegresaber.e-monsite.com/pages/biopolitique.html.
4 Warin, "La flamme d'une chandelle."

5 Warin, "La flamme d'une chandelle."

6 Nancy, "La sindrome biopolitica," p. 58.

7 Nancy, "La sindrome biopolitica," p. 60.

8 P. F. d'Arcais, "Gli inganni di Foucault," *MicroMega*, 8 (2020): 4–33, here p. 30.

9 Galli, "Il doppio volto della biopolitica," pp. 104–5.

10 Galli, "Il doppio volto della biopolitica," pp. 104–5.

11 M. Foucault, "Nietzsche, Genealogy, History," in his *Language, Counter-Memory, Practice: Selected Essays and Interviews*, ed. by D. F. Bouchard. Ithaca: Cornell University Press, 1977, pp. 152–3.

12 M. Foucault, *The Birth of the Clinic: An Archaeology of Medical Perception*, trans. by A. M. Sheridan. London: Routledge, 2003, p. xvi.

13 Regarding the intensely historical character of Foucault's philosophy, see M. Potte-Bonneville, *Michel Foucault: L'inquiétude de l'histoire*. Paris: PUF, 2004 and especially the excellent book by J. Revel, *Foucault avec Merleau-Ponty*. Paris: Vrin, 2015 – where, curiously, she argues that I supposedly "dehistoricized" Foucault (p. 209; she makes the same claim in "Identità, natura, vita: Tre decostruzioni biopolitiche," in M. Galzigna, ed., *Foucault, oggi*. Milan: Feltrinelli, 2008, pp. 134–49).

14 *The Chomsky–Foucault Debate on Human Nature*. New York: New Press, 2006, p. 6.

15 *The Chomsky–Foucault Debate*, p. 29.

16 Foucault, "Nietzsche, Genealogy, History," p. 154.

17 M. Foucault, "Return to History" [1972], trans. by R. Hurley, in *Essential Works of Foucault 1954–1984*, vol. 2: *Aesthetics, Method, and Epistemology*, ed. by James D. Faubion. New York: New Press, 1998, pp. 419–32, here 431. Text based on a transcription reviewed by Foucault of a paper originally presented at Keio University, October 9, 1970.

18 M. Foucault, "The Crisis of Medicine or the Crisis of Antimedicine?" trans. by E. C. Knowlton, Jr., William J. King, and Clare O'Farrell. *Foucault Studies*, 1 (2004): 5–19, here p. 11. DOI: https://doi.org/10.22439/fs.v0i1.562.

19 M. Foucault, *History of Sexuality*, vol. 1: *Introduction (The Will to Knowledge)*, trans. by R. Furley. New York: Pantheon Books, 1978, p. 143, translation slightly modified.

20 M. Foucault, "Bio-History and Bio-Politics" [1994], trans. by Richard A. Lynch. *Foucault Studies*, 18 (2014): 128–30, here p. 129. DOI: https://doi.org/10.22439/fs.v0i18.4655.

21 Foucault, *History of Sexuality*, vol. 1, p. 143.

22 M. Foucault, *Society Must Be Defended: Lectures at the Collège*

de France, 1975–76, trans. by D. Macey. New York: Picador, pp. 55–6 (lecture of 21 January 1976).

23 Foucault, *Society Must Be Defended*, pp. 173–4 (lecture of 25 February 1976).

24 Foucault, *Society Must Be Defended*, pp. 61–2 (lecture of 21 January 1976).

25 Foucault, *Society Must Be Defended*, p. 260 (lecture of 17 March 1976).

26 M. Foucault, *Security, Territory, Population: Lectures at the Collège de France 1977–1978*, trans. by Gr. Burchell. Basingstoke: Macmillan, 2007, pp. 2–3 (lecture of 11 January 1978).

27 Michel Foucault, *Security, Territory, Population: Lectures at the Collège de France 1977–1978*, translated by G. Burchell. Basingstoke: Macmillan, 2007, p. 3 (lecture of 11 January 1978).

28 Foucault, *Security, Territory, Population*, p. 1 (lecture of 11 January 1978).

29 See the editor's note (pp. 273ff.) in the Italian translation of Foucault, *Security, Territory, Population* – a volume edited by M. Senellart (Milan: Feltrinelli, 2005). On the government of life, see S. Chignola, *Foucault oltre Foucault: Una politica della filosofia*. Rome: Deriveapprodi, 2004.

30 See M. Foucault, "La pensée du dehors," *Critique*, 229 (1966). On the concept of "outside" in Foucault, see also R. Esposito, *A Philosophy for Europe: From the Outside*, trans. by Z. Hanafi, Cambridge: Polity, 2018 pp. 131ff. and B. Karsenti, *La politica del "fuori": Una lettura dei corsi di Foucault al Collège de France, 1977–1979*, in S. Chignola, ed., *Governare la vita: Un seminario sui Corsi di Michel Foucault al Collège de France, 1977–1979*. Verona: Ombre Corte, 2006, pp. 71–90.

31 M. Foucault, *The Archaeology of Knowledge and the Discourse on Language*, trans. by A. M. Sheridan Smith. New York: Pantheo, 1972, p. 121.

32 Foucault, *The Archaeology of Knowledge*, p. 122.

33 Foucault, *Security, Territory, Population*, p. 116 (lecture of 8 February 1978).

34 Foucault, *Security, Territory, Population*, p. 116 (lecture of 8 February 1978).

35 Foucault, *Security, Territory, Population*, p. 120 (lecture of 8 February 1978).

36 Foucault, *Security, Territory, Population*, p. 248 (lecture of March 8, 1978).

37 M. Foucault, *The Birth of Biopolitics: Lectures at the Collège*

de France, 1978–1979, trans. by G. Burchell. Basingstoke: Macmillan, 2008 p. 22 (lecture of January 10, 1979).

38 Foucault, *The Birth of Biopolitics*, p. 13 (lecture of January 10, 1979).

39 Foucault, *The Birth of Biopolitics*, p. 17 (lecture of January 10, 1979).

40 Foucault, *The Birth of Biopolitics*, p. 283 (lecture of March 28, 1979).

41 Foucault, *The Birth of Biopolitics*, p. 64 (lecture of January 24, 1979).

42 Foucault, *The Birth of Biopolitics*, p. 69 (lecture of January 24, 1979).

43 On neoliberal anthropology, see the book by M. De Carolis, *Il rovescio della libertà: Tramonto del neo-liberalismo e disagio della libertà*. Macerata: Quodlibet, 2017; and V. Lemm and M. Vatter, eds., *The Government of Life: Foucault, Biopolitics, and Neoliberalism*. New York: Fordham, 2014.

44 Foucault, *The Birth of Biopolitics*, p. 293 (lecture of April 4, 1979).

45 Foucault, *The Birth of Biopolitics*, p. 302 (lecture of April 4, 1979).

46 See T. Lemke, *Biopolitik zur Einführung*. Hamburg: Iunius Verlag, 2007.

47 See N. Rose, *The Politics of Life Itself: Biomedicine, Power, and Subjectivity in the Twenty-First Century*. Princeton: Princeton University Press, 2007.

48 D. Fassin, *La vie: Mode d'emploi critique*. Paris: Seuil, 2018, p. 110 (ch. 3).

49 Fassin, *La Vie*, p. 91 (ch. 2).

50 M. Foucault, *The Punitive Society: Lectures at the Collège de France 1972–1973*, trans. by G. Burchell. Basingstoke: Macmillan, 2015, p. 209 (Lecture of March 21, 1973).

51 M. Foucault, *Psychiatric Power: Lectures at the Collège de France, 1973–1974*, trans. by G. Burchell. Basingstoke: Macmillan, 2006, p. 15 (lecture of November 7, 1973).

52 See E. Goffman, *Asylums: Essays on the Social Situation of Mental Patients and Other Inmates*. Garden City, NY: Anchor Books, 1961.

53 Foucault, *The Birth of Biopolitics*, p. 163 (lecture of February 21, 1979).

54 Foucault, *The Birth of Biopolitics*, p. 167 (lecture of February 21, 1979).

55 Foucault, *The Birth of Biopolitics*, p. 170 (lecture of February 21, 1979).

56 Foucault, *The Birth of Biopolitics*, p. 170 (lecture of February 21, 1979).
57 Foucault, *The Birth of Biopolitics*, p. 174 (lecture of February 21, 1979).
58 Foucault, *The Birth of Biopolitics*, pp. 175, 159–160, 176, 178, and 159–179 passim (the whole lecture 7, of February 21, 1979).
59 I developed this theme in R. Esposito, *Instituting Thought: Three Paradigms of Political Ontology*, trans. by M. W. Epstein. Cambridge: Polity, 2021, pp. 145ff. See also *Discipline filosofiche*, 2 (2019) – a special issue on the institution entitled *Il problema dell'istituzione: Prospettive ontologiche, antropologiche e giuridico-politiche* and edited by E. Lisciani-Petrini and M. Adinolfi. Finally, from a perspective close to the one presented here, see F. Marchesi, "La seconda vita della biopolitica: Dal corpo come eccedenza all'istituzione della vita, 1995–2020," *Teoria*, 41.2 (2021): 51–76.

Notes to Chapter 4

1 See e.g. P. Caspar, *L'individuation des êtres: Aristote, Leibniz et l'immunologie contemporaine*. Paris: Léthielleux, 1985; E. D. Carosella and T. Pradeu, *L'identité, la part de l'autre: Immunologie et philosophie*. Paris: Odile Jacob, 2010; A. D. Napier, "Non self help: How Immunology might reframe the Enlightenment," *Cultural Anthropology*, 27 (2012): 122–137; W. Anderson, "Getting ahead of one's self: The common culture of immunology and philosophy," *Isis*, 105 (2014): 606–16; W. Anderson, "Philosophy of immunology," in *The Stanford Encyclopedia of Philosophy*, 2016. https://plato.stanford.edu/entries/immunology; T. Pradeu, *Philosophy of Immunology*. Cambridge: Cambridge University Press, 2019.
2 M. Heidegger, "The age of the world picture," in his *Off the Beaten Track*, ed. and trans. by J. Young and K. Haynes. Cambridge: Cambridge University Press: 2002, 57–85, here p. 66.
3 Heidegger, "The age of the world picture," p. 75.
4 Heidegger, "The age of the world picture," p. 81.
5 Heidegger, "The age of the world picture," p. 82.
6 Heidegger, "The age of the world picture," p. 84.
7 F. Nietzsche, *Thus Spoke Zatathustra: A Book for All or None*, trans. by A. del Caro. Cambridge: Cambridge University Press, 2006, p. 89.

 8 F. Nietzsche, *The Gay Science, with a Prelude in Rhymes and an Appendix of Songs*, trans. with commentary by Walter Kaufmann. New York: Vintage, 1974, p. 291 (Book 5, §349).

 9 F. Nietzsche, *Human, All Too Human: A Book for the Free Spirits*, trans. by R. J. Hollingdale. Cambridge: Cambridge University Press, 1996, p. 376 (2.2, Aphorism 275,"The age of Cyclopean building").

10 Nietzsche, *Human, All Too Human*, p. 113 (1.5, Aphorism 235, "Genius and the ideal state in conflict").

11 F. Nietzsche, *Daybreak: Thoughts on the Prejudices of Morality*, ed. by Maudemarie Clark and Brian Leiter, trans. by R. J. Hollingdale. Cambridge: Cambridge University Press, 1997, p. 33 (Book 1, Aphorism 52, "Where are the new physicians of the soul?").

12 F. Nietzsche, *The Genealogy of Morals*, trans. by Horace B. Samuel. Mineola, NY: Dover Publications, 2003 [1913], p. 91 (Essay 3, Aphorism 15).

13 F. Nietzsche, *Frammenti postumi (1885–1887)*, in *Opere* (22 vols), vol. 8.1. Milan: Adelphi, 1971, p. 289, trans. from the Italian.

14 Nietzsche, *The Gay Science*, pp. 176–177 (Book 3, §120).

15 Nietzsche, *The Gay Science*, p. 177 (Book 3, §120).

16 Nietzsche, *The Gay Science*, p. 346 (Book 5, §382).

17 Nietzsche, *Human, All Too Human*, p. 107 (1.5, Aphorism 224, "Ennoblement through degeneration").

18 Nietzsche, *Human, All Too Human*, p. 208 (1.5, Aphorism 224, "Ennoblement through degeneration").

19 S. Freud, *The Future of an Illusion* [1927], in S. Freud, *Civilization, Society and Religion, Group Psychology, Civilization and Its Discontents, and Other Works*, vol. 12 of *The Pelican Freud Library*, ed. by A. Dickson, trans. by J. Strachey. Harmondsworth: Penguin Books, 1987, p. 227 (ch. 8).

20 S. Freud, "Freud's Letter to Einstein," in his "Why war?" [1933], in S. Freud, *Civilization, Society and Religion, Group Psychology, Civilization and Its Discontents, and Other Works*, vol. 12 of *The Pelican Freud Library*, ed. by A. Dickson, trans. by J. Strachey. Penguin Books: Harmondsworth, 1987, p. 361.

21 Freud, *Civilization and Its Discontents*, p. 338 (ch. 8).

22 See N. Elias, *Wandlungen des Verhaltens in den weltlichen Oberschichten des Abendlande*, vol. 1: *Changes in the Behavior of the Secular Upper Classes in the West*, trans. by E. Jephcott (with some notes and corrections by the author), rev. edn, ed. by

E. Dunning, J. Goudsblom, and S. Mennell. Oxford: Blackwell Publishers, 2000.

23	Freud, *Civilization and Its Discontents*, p. 338 (ch. 8).

24	Freud, *Civilization and Its Discontents*, p. 314 (ch. 6).

25	S. Freud, *Civilization and Its Discontents*, p. 305 (ch. 5).

26	S. Freud, *Totem and Taboo: Some Points of Agreement between the Mental Lives of Savages and Neurotics* [1913], in vol. 13 of *The Standard Edition of the Complete Psychological Works of Sigmund Freud*, trans. by J. Strachey. London: Hogarth Press, 1958, pp. 141–142.

27	Freud, *Totem and Taboo*, p. 143.

28	Freud, *Totem and Taboo*, p. 143.

29	R. Girard, *Violence and the Sacred*, trans. by P. Gregory. London: Continuum, 2005, p. 273.

30	Girard, *Violence and the Sacred*, p. 31.

31	Girard, *Violence and the Sacred*, p. 305; translation modified on the basis of the French original: *La peste nous introduit déjà dans le climat de la médecine microbienne dans le monde moderne.*

32	Girard, *Violence and the Sacred*, p. 23.

33	Girard, *Violence and the Sacred*, p. 305.

34	Girard, *Violence and the Sacred*, p. 305.

35	Girard, *Violence and the Sacred*, p. 305.

36	R. Girard, *Things Hidden Since the Foundation of the World*, trans. by S. Bann and M. Metteer. London: Bloomsbury Academic, 2016, p. 23.

37	Girard, *Things Hidden Since the Foundation of the World*, p. 245.

38	Girard, *Things Hidden Since the Foundation of the World*, p. 247.

39	Girard, *Things Hidden Since the Foundation of the World*, pp. 240–150.

40	N. Luhmann, *Social Systems*, trans. by J. Bednarz and D. Baecker. Stanford, CA: Stanford University Press, 1995, p. 383.

41	Luhmann, *Social Systems*, p. 383.

42	N. Luhmann, "How is social order possible?" Ch. 2 in his *The Making of Meaning: From the Individual to Social Structure: Selections from Works on Semantics and Social Structure*, ed. by C. Morgner, trans. by M. Hiley, C. Morgner, and M. King. New York: Oxford University Press, 2022, pp. 84–178. Online edn, Oxford Academic, 21 Apr. 2022. DOI: https://doi.org/10.1093/oso/9780190945992.001.0001.

43	Luhmann, *Social Systems*, p. 371.

44	Luhmann, *Social Systems*, p. 170.

45 Luhmann, *Social Systems*, pp. 171–2.
46 N. Luhmann, "The autopoiesis of social systems," in *Sociocybernetic Paradoxes: Observation, Control and Evolution of Self-Steering Systems*, ed. by Felix Geyer and J. van der Zouwen. London: SAGE, 1986, 176–205, here p. 182. On the relationship between autopoiesis and immunology, see W. S. Guerra Filho, *"Luhmann and immunology and autopoiesis," in Luhmann Observed: Radical Theoretical Encounters*. London: Palgrave MacMillan, 2013, pp. 227–42; H. Richter, "Beyond the 'other' as constitutive outside: The politics of immunity in Roberto Esposito and Niklas Luhmann," in *European Journal of Political Theory*, 18.2 (2016): 1–22; S. Grampp and O. Moskatova, "Medien der Immunität. Politiken und Praktiken von Schutz und Ansteckung," *H/Soz/Kult*, 24 August 2020. https://www.hsozkult.de/searching/id/event-93048?language=de.
47 Luhmann, "The autopoiesis of social systems," p. 185.
48 Luhmann, *Social Systems*, pp. 373–4.
49 Luhmann, *Social Systems*, p. 375.
50 Luhmann, *Social Systems*, p. 375.
51 Luhmann, *Social Systems*, p. 375.
52 Luhmann, *Social Systems*, p. 389.
53 Luhmann, *Social Systems*, p. 394.
54 Luhmann, *Social Systems*, p. 395.
55 N. Luhmann, *La differenziazione del diritto: Contributi alla sociologia e alla teoria del diritto*. Bologna: il Mulino, 1990, p. 58; trans. from the Italian. (Original publication: N. Luhmann, *Ausdifferenzierung des Rechts: Beiträge zur Rechtssoziologie und Rechtstheorie*. Suhrkamp: Frankfurt am Mein, 1981.)
56 J. Derrida, "Faith and knowledge: The two sources of 'religion' at the limits of reason alone," in his *Acts of Religion*, ed. by G. Anidjar. New York: Routledge, 2002 [1998], 40–101, here p. 88 (§41).
57 See S. Regazzoni, *Derrida: Biopolitica e democrazia*. Genova: il Nuovo Melangolo, 2012, pp. 65ff; A. Marchente, "Autoimmunità: Tra biopolitica e decostruzione," *Esercizi filosofici*, 9 (2014): 79–97.
58 J. Derrida, *Specters of Marx: The State of the Debt, the Work of Mourning, and the New International*, trans. by P. Kamuf. New York: Routledge, 1994, p. 177.
59 J. Derrida, "To Speculate: On Freud," in his *The Post Card: From Socrates to Freud and Beyond*, trans. by A. Bass. Chicago, IL: University of Chicago Press, 1987, pp. 1–256, here p. 361.
60 Derrida, "Faith and knowledge, p. 80 (§37, n. 27).

61 Derrida, "Faith and knowledge," p. 82 (§37).
62 See J. H. Miller, "Derrida's politics of autoimmunity," *Discourse*, 30 (2008): 208–25; F. Evans, "Derrida and auto-immunity of democracy," *Journal of Speculative Philosophy*, 3 (2016): 303–15; P. Mitchell, "Contagion, virology, autoim-munity: Derrida's rethoric of contamination," in *Parallax*, 23 (2017): 77–93; E. Timár, "Derrida's error and immunology," *Oxford Literary Review*, 1 (2017): 65–81; R. Mendoza de Jesús, "Another life: Democracy, suicide, ipseity, autoimmun-ity," *Enrahonar: An International Journal of Theoretical and Practical Reason*, 66 (2021): 15–35; C. Wolfe, "(Auto)immu-nity in Esposito e Derrida," in T. Rayan and A. Calcagno, *New Directions in Biophilosophy*. Edinburgh: Edinburgh University Press, 2021.
63 Derrida, "Faith and knowledge," p. 80 (§37).
64 J. Derrida, "Autoimmunity: Real and symbolic suicides," in G. Borradori, *Philosophy in a Time of Terror: Dialogues with Jurgen Habermas and Jacques Derrida*. Chicago, IL: University of Chicago Press, 2013, p. 99.
65 Derrida, "Faith and knowledge," p. 89 (§42).
66 Derrida, "Faith and knowledge," p. 87 (§40).
67 P. Sloterdijk, *Spheres*, vol. 1: *Bubbles: Microspherology*, trans. by W. Hoban. Cambridge, MA: MIT Press, 2011, p. 28.
68 P. Sloterdijk, *You Must Change Your Life*, trans. by W. Hoban. Cambridge: Polity, 2013, p. 10.
69 Sloterdijk, *You Must Change Your Life*, p. 11.
70 Sloterdijk, *Spheres*, p. 25. On Peter Sloterdijk, see A. Lucci, *Il limite delle sfere. Saggio su Peter Sloterdijk*. Bulzoni, Rome, 2011; W. Schinkel and L. Noordegraaf-Eelens (eds.), *In Medias Res. Peter Sloterdijk's Spherological Poetics of Being*. Amsterdam: University Press, 2011; Mutsaers, *Immunological Discourse in Political Philosophy*, pp. 75ff.
71 Peter Sloterdijk, *In the World Interior of Capital: For a Philosophical Theory of Globalization*. Cambridge: Polity, 2013, p. 92 (Ch. 16, "Between Justifications and Assurances: On Terran and Maritime Thought").
72 Sloterdijk, *In the World Interior of Capital*, p. 86 (Ch. 16, "Between justifications and assurances: On terran and maritime thought").
73 Sloterdijk, *You Must Change Your Life*, p. 451.
74 Sloterdijk, *You Must Change Your Life*, pp. 451–452.

Notes to Chapter 5

1 Patrick Zylberman, *Tempêtes microbiennes: Essai sur la politique sanitaire dans le monde transatlantique*. Paris: Gallimard, 2013, p. 24.
2 J.-P. Dupuy, *Pour un catastrophisme éclairé: Quand l'impossible est certain*. Paris: Seuil, 2004, p. 180, as quoted in Zylberman, *Tempêtes microbiennes*, p. 39.
3 Zylberman, *Tempêtes microbiennes*, p. 40.
4 R. Preston, *The Cobra Event*. New York: Ballantine Books, 1997. Preston's later novels – *The Hot Zone: The Terrifying True Story of the Origins of the Ebola Virus*. New York: Anchor Books, 1995; and *The Demon in the Freezer*. New York: Random House, 2000 – were equally successful.
5 L. Garret, *The Coming Plague: Newly Emerging Diseases in a World Out of Balance*. New York: Farrar, Straus & Giroux, 1994; and Garret, *Betrayal of Trust. The Collapse of Global Public Health*. Oxford: Oxford University Press, 2000.
6 Note how they are described by R. Sunstein, director of the Office of Information and Regulatory Affairs, in his *Worst-Case Scenario*. Cambridge, MA: Harvard University Press, 2009. Regarding the underlying "logic of the worst," see C. Rosset, *La logique du pire. Éléments pour une philosophie tragique*. Paris: PUF, 1971, as well as J. Whitman, ed., *Politics of Emergent and Resurgent Infectious Diseases*. Basingstoke: Macmillan, 2000; D. Rosner and G. Markowitz, *Are We Ready? Public Health since 9/11*. Berkeley: University of California Press, 2006; O. Borraz, *Les politiques du risque*. Paris: Presses de Science Po, 2008.
7 J. Habermas and K. Günther, "Kein Grundrecht gilt grenzenlos," *Die Zeit*, May 2020.
8 R. Birnbaum and G. Ismar, "Schaüble will dem Schutz des Lebens nicht alles unterordnen," *Tagesspiel*, April 26, 2020. https://www.tagesspiegel.de/politik/bundestagspraesident-zur-corona-krise-schaeuble-will-dem-schutz-des-lebens-nicht-alles-unterordnen/25770466.html. Original text: "Grundrechte beschränken sich gegenseitig. Wenn es überhaupt einen absoluten Wert in unserem Grundgesetz gibt, dann ist das die Würde des Menschen. Die ist unantastbar. Aber sie schließt nicht aus, dass wir sterben müssen."
9 See J. Habermas, *Die Zukunft der menschlichen Natur: Auf dem Weg zur liberalen Eugenetik*. Frankfurt am Mein: Suhrkamp, 2001.

10 On the relationship between freedom and health, see C. Iannello, *Salute e libertà: Il fondamentale diritto all'autodeterminazione individuale*, Editoriale scientifica. Naples, 2020; C. Ocone, *Salute o libertà: Un dilemma storico-filosofico*. Soveria Mannelli: Rubbettino, 2021.

11 See the still useful book by Ph. Bobbitt and G. Calabresi, *Tragic Choices*, Norton & Company, New York 1978; and the Italian edition *Scelte tragiche*, Giuffrè, Milano 2006, with a preface by S. Rodotà.

12 For the discussion in Italy, see G. Agamben, *A che punto siamo? L'epidemia come politica*. Macerata: Quodlibet, 2020; G. Zagrebelsky, "Non è l'emergenza che mina la democrazi:. Il pericolo è l'eccezione," *La Repubblica*, July 29, 2020; C. Galli, "Epidemia tra norma ed eccezione," April 9, 2020. https://www.iisf.it/index.php/progetti/diario-della-crisi/carlo-galli-epidemia-tra-norma-ed-eccezione.html.

13 See C. Schmitt, *Dictatorship*, trans. by M. Hoelzl and G. Ward. Cambridge: Polity, 2014.

14 S. Romano, "Sui decreti-legge e lo stato di assedio in occasione del terremoto di Messina e di Reggio Calabria," *Rivista di diritto pubblico*, 1909, p. 289 (italics added). https://messinacitta.wordpress.com/2020/03/08/santi-romano-articolo-sui-decreti-legge-e-lo-stato-di-assedio-in-occasione-del-terremoto-di-messina-e-di-reggio-calabria-in-rivista-di-diritto-pubblico-e-della-pubblica-amministrazione-in-italia.

15 Romano, "Sui decreti-legge," pp. 297–8.

16 Romano, "Sui decreti-legge," p. 294.

17 On the complex relationship between politics and science, see the book on Weber by M. Cacciari, *Il lavoro dello spirito*. Milan: Adelphi, 2020. For an interesting parallel between our crisis and that of the Weimer Republic, with reference to the immune paradigm, see F. Serra di Cassano, *R-esistere: Dal pathos della "Kultur" al paradigma immunitario: Thomas Mann e le tensioni della modernità*. Naples: Bibliopolis, 2021.

18 On the government of experts, see D. Di Cesare's timely remarks in her *Virus sovrano: L'asfissia capitalistica*. Turin: Bollati Boringhieri, 2020, with an explicit reference to the immune paradigm. Also on this subject, see A. Martone, *NoCity: Paura e democrazia nell'età globale*. Rome: Castelvecchi, 2021, pp. 107ff.

19 See C. J. Bickerton and C. Invernizzi Accetti, *Technopopulism: The New Logic of Democratic Politics*. Oxford: Oxford University Press, 2021.

20 A. Mantovani, *Il fuoco interiore: Il sistema immunitario e l'origine delle malattie*. Milan: Mondadori, 2021.
21 D. C. Fajgenbaum, L. Rénia, L. F. P. Ng, and C. H. June, "Cytokine storm," *New England Journal of Medicine*, 383 (2020): 2255–73.
22 M. Z. Tay, C. M. Poh and P. A. MacAry, "The trinity of Covid-19: Immunity, inflammation and intervention," *Nature Reviews Immunology*, 20 (2020): 363–74.
23 See P. Ehrlich and J. Morgenroth, "Über Hämolysine V: Mitteilung," *Berliner Klinische Wochenschrift*, 38 (1901): 251–7. On this topic, see S. Avrameas, "Natural autoantibodies: From 'horror autotoxicus' to 'gnothi seauton', *Immunology Today*, 12 (1991, pp. 154–9; A. M. Silverstein, "Autoimmunity versus horror autotoxicus: The struggle for recognition," *Nature Immunology*, 2 (2001): 279–81; S. Herbrechter and M. Jamieson, eds., *Autoimmunities*, special issue of *Parallax*, 23 (2017).
24 See A. Viola, *Danzare nella tempesta: Viaggio nella fragile perfezione del sistema immunitario*. Milan: Feltrinelli, 2021.
25 See L. Margulis, *Symbiosis in Cell Evolution*. New York: Freeman, 1981; S. F. Gilbert, J. Sapp, and A. I. Tauber, "A symbiotic way of life: We have never been Individuals," *Quarterly Review of Biology*, 87 (2012): 325–41; E. Muraille, "Redefining the immune system as a social interface for cooperative process," *PLoS Pathogens*, 9 (2013). https://journals.plos.org/plospathogens/article?id=10.1371/journal. ppat.1003203; Y. Belkaid and O. J. Harrison, "Homeostatic immunity and the microbiota," in *Immunity*, 46 (2017): 562–76; G. Eberl, "A new vision of immunity: Homeostasis of the superorganism," in *Mucosal Immunology*, 3 (2010): 450–60.
26 On the misuse of the war metaphor for Covid-19, see E. Martinez-Brawley and E. Gualda, "Transnational social implications of the use of the 'war metaphor' concerning coronavirus: A bird's eye view," *Culture e Studi del Sociale*, 5 (2020): 259–72.
27 Frank Macfarlane Burnet, *The Integrity of the Body: A Discussion of Modern Immunological Ideas*. Cambridge, MA: Harvard University Press, 1962, p. 68. See also Frank Macfarlane Burnet, *Self and Not-Self: Cellular Immunology*. London: Cambridge University Press, 1969.
28 See E. M. Lance, P. B. Medawar, and E. Simpson, *An Introduction to Immunology*. London: Wildwood House, 1977.
29 Niels Kaj Jerne, "Toward a network theory of the immune system," *Annales de l'Institut Pasteur*, 125 (1974): 373–89, here 381.

30 Alfred I. Tauber, *The Immune Self: Theory or Metaphor?* Cambridge: Cambridge University Press, 1997, p. 196.

31 S. Lidgard and L. K. Nyhart, "The work of biological individuality: Concepts and contexts," in *Biological Individuality: Integrating Scientific, Philosophical, and Historical Perspectives*, ed. by S. Lidgard and L. K. Nyhart, Chicago, IL: University of Chicago Press, 2017, pp. 17–62; A. Guay and T. Pradeu, *Individuals across the Sciences*. New York: Oxford University Press, 2016.

32 See T. Martin, ed., *Le tout et les parties dans les systèmes naturels*. Paris: Vuibert, 2007; E. D. Carosella and T. Pradeu, *L'identité, la part de l'autre: Immunologie et philosophie*. Paris: Odile Jacob, 2010; T. Pradeu, *Les limites du soi: immunologie et identité biologique*, Paris: Press Universitaires de Montréal, 2009.

33 See L. Chiu, T. Bazin, M. E. Truchetet, T. Schaeverbeke, L. Delhaes, and T. Pradeu, "Protective microbiota: From localized to long-reaching co-immunity," *Front Immunology*, 8 (2017). https://www.frontiersin.org/articles/10.3389/fimmu.2017.01 678/ full.

34 For more on this idea, see P. Vineis, *Salute senza confini: Le epidemie della globalizzazione*. Turin: Codice, 2020.

35 See *Raggiungeremo mai l'immunità di gregge?* March 19, 2021, which picks up on an article from *Nature*. https://www.ilposgi ungeremo-mai-limmunita-di-gregge.

36 For an original interpretation of community in territories, see the recent work by A. Bonomi, *Oltre le mura dell'impresa: Vivere, abitare, lavorare nelle piattaforme territoriali*. Rome: DeriveApprodi, 2021.